About the author

Juliette de Baïracli Levy is a world-wide authority on the natural rearing of animals and a pioneer in the field of their treatment by herbal medicine. She has proved over many years that her treatments and diets for animals are safe and effective and she is a renowned breeder of Turkuman Afghan hounds. She has cared for and loved cats all through her long and much-travelled life. As well as being a botanist and practical herbalist, she is also a soil doctor and anthologist of gypsy lore. Born in Manchester, of Turkish parentage, Juliette de Baïracli Levy now lives in Greece.

'I have found several herbals helpful but the herbalist I respect most is Juliette de Baïracli Levy, whose advice seems to me most grounded in experience with animals, people and her own children. She is also familiar with the medicines of nomadic people . . . and thus draws from other, older cultures. Moreover she seems to be a true healer with humility and love for people. I would advise anyone interested in herbs to go directly to her books.' From *An Herbal Sampler* by Elaine Goldman Gill, renowned American herbalist.

CATS – NATURALLY
Natural Rearing for Healthier Cats
Juliette de Baïracli Levy

Illustrated by Linda Herd

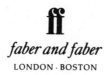

faber and faber
LONDON · BOSTON

First published in 1991
by Faber and Faber Limited
3 Queen Square, London WC1N 3AU

Photoset by Parker Typesetting Service, Leicester
Printed in Great Britain by Cox & Wyman Ltd, Reading, Berkshire

Juliette de Baïracli Levy is hereby identified as author of
this work in accordance with Section 77 of the Copyright,
Designs and Patents Act 1988

A CIP record for this book
is available from the British Library.

ISBN 0–571–16231–2

2 4 6 8 10 9 7 5 3 1

To a long-time and beloved friend, Helen Scott Nearing, who appreciates cats, and to *Pamouk* (Turkish for 'cotton'), our white cat, the first 'domestic' cat to share with us our nature life in England's New Forest.

'. . . it is cat, which yet keeps a large part of its heart and soul untameable'.

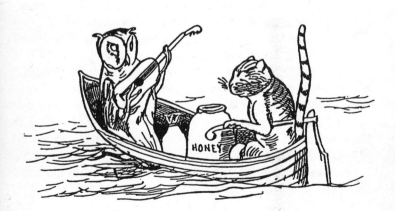

IMPORTANT NOTE FOR READERS IN GREAT BRITAIN

In recent years, the natural habitat of many wild plants has disappeared and some herbs have become rare in the wild because of building developments, intensive farming, and other pressures on land use.

In an effort to prevent these rare plants from extinction, the Wildlife and Countryside Act 1981 and its Variation of Schedule Order 1988 make it an offence for any unauthorized person to pick, uproot, destroy or offer for sale almost a hundred wild plants in Great Britain.

It is also an offence for an unauthorized person to *uproot any wild plant*, whether or not it is on the protected list.

The author strongly advises readers to grow their own herbs or obtain dried herbs from health food shops.

The Wildlife and Countryside Act 1981 and the Wildlife and Countryside Act (Variation of Schedule) Order 1988 can be obtained through HMSO bookshops. Alternatively, a list of the fully protected plant species can be obtained from the Department of the Environment, Tollgate House, Houlton Street, Bristol, BS2 9DJ.

Readers in countries other than Great Britain should check local regulations before gathering flowers in the wild.

Contents

Country cats, Cat play, Climbing cats, Modern cat
life, Climbing needs, Training, Cat claws,
De-clawing, Scratching places, Raising kittens, Size of
litters, Unwanted kittens, Training of kittens,
Obedience, Removing kittens from their mother,
Naming a kitten, Survival of cats, Health hazards,
Natural life for cats, Wild and feral cats, Exercise for
town cats, Entertainment for cats, Cat dens, Fleas,
Bathing

Vegetarian foods, Size of feeds, Cats and birds, Fresh
foods, Herbs, Diet for health, Flesh foods, Fish,
Bones, Milk, Cheese, Cereals, Other foods for cats,
Oil for cats, 'Pet foods', Raw foods, Legumes, Natural
Rearing Diets, NR Diet for kittens, Weaning, NR Diet
for adult cats

Acknowledgements

The author would like to thank Faber and Faber Ltd and Harcourt Brace Jovanovich Inc. for permission to quote from 'The Naming of Cats', *Old Possum's Book of Practical Cats*, T. S. Eliot, 1939.

Foreword

World wide today there is a cat cult.

We know that the ancient Egyptians worshipped cats. Presentday, it is reckoned that three cats are kept for every dog. Space problems may be the reason for this, though the character of the domestic cat also contributes to popularity, for the cat is affectionate, clever, amusing and resourceful. And cats are also very useful catchers of house mice, which nowadays are a menace world wide.

Cats – Naturally will be of interest to all cat-lovers because it is something different among cat books for it adapts much esteemed herbal medicine for the needs of cats. The author has behind her herbal work a half century of experience and success. Her veterinary herbal books have been translated into many languages.

Prevention of ailments through natural diet is an important feature of this book. Detailed Natural Rearing Diets to give and maintain good health are provided. The reader will be intrigued by the variety of natural foods which have been proved acceptable to the cat, as felines have many vegetarian inclinations from sweet-corn to a mixture of berries.

This book also has its lighter side. Verses from cat poems grace the text, and there is a list of hundreds of cat names, mostly classified by colour, collected from many lands, to amuse the reader and provide inspiration when a new kitten needs a name.

FOREWORD

The beautiful black-and-white illustrations by Linda Herd will give much additional pleasure to the readers of *Cats – Naturally*. Finally, my thanks to Sarah Gleadell for all her excellent and clever ideas for this book; also many thanks to Barbara Ellis for her very skilled and caring editing.

1

Introduction

The domestic cat, likewise the domestic dog, and the (wild) owl were put on earth by God to protect mankind. All three of these creatures have the ability to see in the dark of night (when man sleeps, and is most defenceless and likely to be harmed).

There are many legends about all three of these helpers. For instance, it is told that when the Ark was ready to sail, carrying to safety from the flood all God's chosen family and all the many non-human creatures (including the cat!) that he had created with such loving care and skill, the Devil thought up an evil plan to destroy the Ark and all its inmates. He cunningly made a creature evil as his plan – the rat – giving it the power to swim well, sight in the darkness and the ability to gnaw through wood. This creation of the Devil was to swim, unseen, to the Ark, and when the Ark was far enough from shore, to gnaw holes beneath the water-line and thus cause it to sink, drowning all within it except the rat, which would swim back to the Devil's protection!

But the dog discovered the hole that the rat was gnawing and the pair of dogs took turns in pressing their noses into the hole until Noah was alerted and repaired the damage. (That is why to this day the dog has a long nose and a wet one!)

The night creatures, cat and owl, then kept watch to ensure that the rats (a pair, as all other inmates of the Ark) did not

gnaw more holes, and the rats were harassed and chased
whenever they were seen outside their hiding places in the
Ark. But for extra trouble the Devil made the rat carrier of the
baneful flea, harmful to this day.

Then there is a legend (a beautiful one) about the cat. This
cat is credited with having saved Muhammad from death

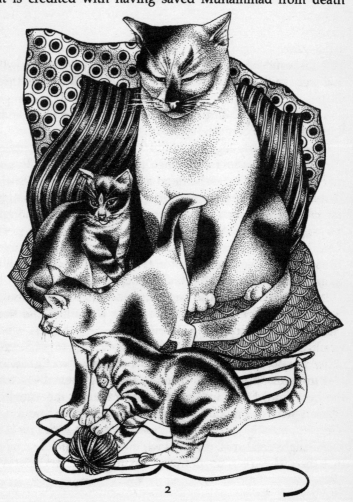

when an evil spirit, in the form of a serpent, climbed unseen up Muhammad's gown and was about to strike at the prophet's heart.

The cat leapt between snake and man, and took the fatal strike instead. The cat died, but Muhammad then put a special blessing on cats: he promised that henceforth all cats should have ten lives. 'Ten lives I will give to you cats as reward for one of you saving my life. One life has already been taken from you by the snake, but nine further lives remain with you. Nine further times death will come to you, but you will survive until you have used up all your nine lives.'

That is why to this day the cat is near worshipped in many Muslim countries and few Muslims will kill a cat.

The Greeks have a different cat belief. They claim that the cat is the chief protector of mankind against all the dangerous nocturnal creatures, among which they include the snake. They say that the cat protected the infant Jesus in the manger, against the rodents and snakes, and therefore Christ later blessed the cat, and to this day the cat is allowed within Greek homes and petted and cared for, whereas the unfortunate dog is kept outdoors only, on a short chain with a miserable wooden box for its dwelling!

The cat belongs to the most noble and most powerful of all the animal families, the feline. Among its kind are the kings of the animal world, in which God must have taken special care and looked upon with well-deserved pride – the great cats: the lions, tigers, panthers, leopards.

And although the domestic cat is by far the smallest of the many cat types, even a young kitten walks with tail upright in dignity, a true example of its much admired and feared race. Of all domestic creatures it is the cat who yet keeps its heart untameable.

Indeed there is a popular book by Richard Taber, *The Wild*

Life of the Domestic Cat, which has had very favourable reviews, including one from the BBC's weekly programme, *Nature Now*.

The American cats and dogs expert and author, Jean Harper, in her interesting book, *The Healthy Cat and Dog Cook-Book* (Sloodic Press, Chicago) tells about the ancient history of cats: 'Cats have been companions of mankind since thousands of years. In Egypt they were considered as sacred symbols, and in Siam they guarded royal palaces.' Those beautiful and clever blue-eyed Siamese cats! Now found world wide and deeply loved by all who have ever owned one.

Cats deserve an honoured place in the human home because, of all the domestic animals, it is the cat which is credited as being chief protector against those evil, dirty and destructive creatures, rats, and their close relatives, mice.

And those dangerous vermin are greatly on the increase nowadays, helped by the enormous amounts of litter which are part of modern living, and by the fact that destructive agro-chemicals have killed off most of nature's wild birds and animals created by God to control rodents, especially the owls, hawks and hedgehogs.

The rat hordes are around, eating or contaminating with their excreta a near half of the world's food supplies. And through their very prevalent fleas they are spreaders of tapeworms and the dreaded bubonic plague.

Therefore, as an anti-rodent measure, *keep a cat*! But keep that cat healthy by the now well-proved successful method of Natural Rearing.

Unfortunately the ailments of the modern cat, similar to the increase in the number of rodents, are increasing daily and that is due to unnatural diet and to unnatural care for ill animals.

Whereas the typical ailments of the feline tribe, the cats, as

4

with the carnivores, the dog, were formerly a mere half dozen, all of them easily curable by fasting and the intake of suitable herbs, herbs which were well known to dogs and cats who sought them out and used them, present-day ailments fill large veterinary books and new pages to cope with ever-new ailments have to be added yearly. Also now, the dread cancer, once unknown to the carnivores and felines, and as yet rarely found among the wild tribes of these species, is widespread and a true menace.

I have not attempted to deal with all these new cat ailments in my chapter on herbal remedies. I have dealt with the more typical ones, all of which, I am thankful to say, are curable without lengthy treatments.

Concerning the keeping of a cat or cats in the human home – and this applies to all domestic animals – I quote appropriate words from the famous American Red Indian chief, Chief Seattle, from his great and inspired speech in defence of his native lands in North America, defence from the destructive inroads made by the white Americans.

His speech, known as 'This Earth is Precious', is indeed more appropriate today than when it was made many years ago.

'What is man without the beasts? If all the beasts were gone, man would die from a great loneliness of spirit. For whatever happens to the beasts soon happens to man. All things are connected.'

I am sure that God, the creator of all, understood this when he put the beasts with such loving care into the Ark.

Jean Harper also aptly writes, 'No picture of the human family hearth is really right without the family cat curled up there and exuding a feeling of warmth and comfort.' (I have also had a pet hedgehog and tortoise sharing my hearth with hounds and cat, all there *in good-natured fellowship*. Thank God for that, and for them: my animal friends.)

5

Doris Lessing, in her beautiful book, *Particularly Cats* (Panther Books), writes deeply about the souls of cats, and what a difference the possession of cats makes to human life. She describes one cat which she could never replace in her heart, a blue Persian cat which helped her in illness, in a way which dogs cannot really do: 'Arrived purring on my bed, and settled down to share my sickness, my food, my pillow, my sleep.'

The American cat expert, Carole C. Wilboum, in her popular column, 'Cat Talk', gives good advice to cat-lovers who are prevented from keeping a cat because of cat allergies, by publishing a note from a reader who overcame this problem very well:

> I thought you'd be interested to know that I used to be deathly allergic to cats. Asthma was my primary problem. But two years ago, Fortune, a tiny kitten, came into my life and I outgrew my allergy. My allergist said I built up the antibodies from constant exposure to cat dander and fur. I now have eight cats and plan to move to a house in the suburbs so we can all stretch out in abundant space. I can't tell you how happy I am that Fortune made it possible for me to be such a cat person.

Cats are also considered to be healers for human disturbed nerves. It is agreed that a purring cat in a bedroom will help a human into sleep far better than any chemical sleeping pill, and stroking cats (or dogs) is widely recognized as being of psychological aid in helping people to relax.

When one truly loves and understands cats, one is likely to write well concerning them. And that certainly applies to the books of T. S. Eliot, loved and kept by all cat-lovers. Perhaps the most famous of his cat writings is his *Old Possum's Book of Practical Cats* (Faber and Faber), on which a great theatrical show, called *Cats*, has been based and has been running in

London for several years. All cat-lovers should read and enjoy 'The Theatre Cat'. Here is the town cat at its most lofty and boastful and amusing best.

2

Raising the Domestic Cat

When planning the raising of our cat or cats, we must keep foremost in our minds the fact that it is the cat which has remained closest to Nature, and that if cats are not allowed to lead at least a fairly natural life they will become miserable and never attain maximum good health; their natures will also become spiteful and, finally, they may well run away. Furthermore, cats are natural creatures of the night, more apt to sleep by day and become active by night. Indeed, they come under the classification of nocturnal. Their sight in the darkness is excellent and it is then that they hunt out and kill their chosen prey, those filthy and destructive creatures, the rodents – rats and mice.

Cats are also killers and eaters of scorpions and they kill the hateful cockroaches, but do not eat them. Therefore try and provide *some* nightlife for domestic cats. If they cannot be allowed to roam free by night, then at least see they can play in a darkened room for a while nightly.

COUNTRY CATS

Of course, if your cat shares a farm life or a country dwelling with you, then its raising is a very simple matter: mostly the cat takes care of itself, both for its food and exercise. Cats are great self-providers.

For the country-living cat one needs to provide the traditional (old-fashioned) cat-door for the cat to enter and leave at will the human dwelling. This cat-door is merely a piece cut out of the door at the base, big enough for the cat to pass through. The piece is then fixed with string and nail to the door from which it has been cut and is fortified, preferably with a spring. The cat soon learns to push open its door when it wants to enter or leave its owner's house. Unfortunately, rats and other cats may also make use of the cat-door! But a good cat will soon take care of them if they dare to enter its owner's house. Nowadays one can easily obtain ready-made cat-flaps which can be fitted to doors. The ultimate in sophistication is the electronic cat-flap which is fitted with a special device: the household cat wears a small collar also containing a matching electronic device. The cat-flap so fitted will admit only the household cat, not unwelcome visitors such as rats, mice or other cats. The electronic device in the cat's collar activates the cat-flap.

The domestic cat, free to come and go and with access to the countryside, hunts down its own food, kills and (usually) eats rodents, young rabbits, lizards, frogs and snakes. Not all cats will eat rodents when they kill them, but mostly they will do so. Sometimes young cats will not kill their prey but just play with them.

Unfortunately, cats also kill young hedgehogs, which charming creatures are true friends of the countryside. Hedgehogs kill entire nests of mice; they kill mice not to eat them but because they realize they are enemies to their chosen

9

food supplies, the wild grains, fruits and nuts of the country-side. Hedgehogs kill mice in the nest, young ones and adult, by rolling on them and crushing them with their body prickles.

The self-hunting country cat requires from its human owners only basic foods such as milk and cereals. I shall enlarge on this in the next chapter, on diet.

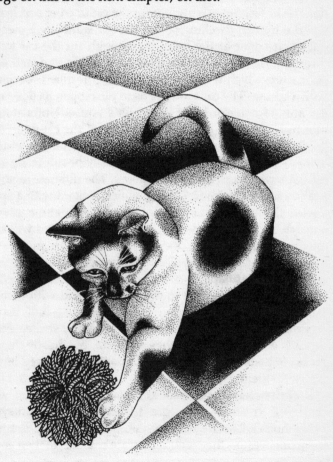

CAT PLAY

Cats are by nature very playful. They love to leap around and to chase after things. If cats are confined to the house, playthings must be provided for them if they are to remain happy and healthy. As we provide balls and sticks for our dogs to retrieve, so likewise we must select favoured playthings for cats. The mouths of cats are not suitable for holding hard things such as heavy balls or sticks. A ball of wool is a more suitable cat plaything.

An American reader of my *Complete Herbal Handbook for the Dog and Cat* sent me a cutting, in colour, from a US magazine featuring an article on cats as pets. The cutting was of attractive pictures of cats at play. One showed a kitten clawing at a woollen pom-pom (small ball) and had the caption: 'Pompoms placed throughout the house can help keep cats happily occupied when owners are away.' Another picture is of a cat leaping after a ping-pong ball and has the caption: 'Pingpong balls (or nerf balls) drive some cats wild!' Cats do indeed love the lightness of a ping-pong ball and the sound of its rattle as it skims across the floor and, unlike the dog, there is no danger of the cat's swallowing such a ball.

The third picture showed a picture of a cat scattering feathers from a feather duster. Feathers give great excitement to a cat, so remember to keep any feathers to use for cat-play when one brings poultry into the kitchen for cooking.

CLIMBING CATS

Cats are also adventurous and skilled climbers, in character the same as the big cats of the feline family. When on a climbing expedition, up aloft on some high tree, leaping from bough to bough, cats are wonderful to watch. Little tigers!

And this resemblance is not only in their skilled and supple movements; their eyes possess 'tiger-light', and their whiskers bristle like those of the big cats.

Here is some advice about climbing cats: if one's cat climbs very high up a tree, either from alarm at being dog-chased, or from a frightening noise, or on a hunting trip after birds or other prey, and it seems unable to descend from a great height, the cat-owner should not panic and go to the expense and trouble of calling the fire service to bring a ladder and rescue the cat as is often done. One can be positive that every cat can descend from any tree-height to which it has climbed, even though it may remain there for a long time, perhaps for several days.

MODERN CAT LIFE

Many cats are never in their lifetime able to hunt prey across countryside, nor climb a tree; they are totally house-confined. This house-confinement mostly applies to town-dwelling cats as their owners do not want to risk the dangers of cat thieves, who sell stolen cats as pets to others, or to be eaten, or to be skinned for their pelts. Town cats also run the risk of poison put down for rodents or by cat-haters, and more frequently the risk of being injured in road accidents.

If cats have to be house-confined, then all I have written about feline love of the dark and of play preferences becomes of special importance if one wants to own a happy and healthy cat. Not only are sessions in the dark needed, but the domestic cat, in common with all the feline tribe, loves the sunlight. To deprive any cat of daily access to sunlight, when available, is truly cruel.

The American author and naturalist, Svevo Brooks, told me that he arranged the windows of a house he built by observing the places around the building under construction where his cats chose to sun themselves. He wanted a warm, sun-filled house and he used sun-bathing cats as a guide for the placing of his windows!

If the apartment where a cat must live is a dark one, the owner may have a large wire cage positioned as an extension outside, leading from a window and secured strongly to the brickwork. In such a cage a cat can take its much-needed sun-bath because cats, in the same way as cattle and other creatures, lick sun-vitamins, especially vitamin A, from their hair during sun-bathing. The cage can also help the cat to enjoy its other love, moonlight-bathing.

Climbing needs

The cat's climbing needs must be provided for in an apartment. This is best done by purchase of a small ladder. For the cat's pleasure, bind the steps of the ladder with strong, webbed cloth, such as is used for floor-cleaning. This will not only make the ladder exercise more easy, it will also provide much-needed claw-exercise scratching places for the cat, who should be taught to do its scratching there by holding the cat and rubbing its feet to and fro on the rough surface. (Then the cat will not use good materials in the apartment for exercising its claws.) Further for the cat's pleasure, make a flat seat on the top of the ladder, placing a cushion there, filled with cotton padding, not plastics material.

Up there on its high seat, the cat – tiger-like – can pose aloft, as it loves to do, and survey all that goes on down below!

TRAINING

In the raising of cats, their training is important. All domestic animals, whether house pets or our ponies and goats outdoors, even our pigeons and poultry, need to be trained, for their happiness as well as their owner's convenience.

The dog is easily trainable and seems to enjoy this (as can be seen in circus dogs who generally perform well and look happy), whereas cats are often difficult to train and need much time and care in this respect: an untrained cat within the home is a nuisance and I personally could never tolerate this. Cats allowed to 'do as they please' knock valuable things off tables and shelves, claw and thus tear or badly scratch, furniture and curtains, steal food, and harm (or even suffocate) human infants by sleeping on top of them for their comfortable warmth.

Dogs are not likely, unless under great stress, to scratch or bite their owners but cats, unless carefully trained, may well bite and scratch humans.

They must be carefully trained in kittenhood to be gentle and not aggressive by a quiet human voice and careful handling, not by harsh words or hitting. Keep hands for fondling and if a cat needs to be punished for some truly bad deed, then use a folded newspaper, not the human hand. *Never* try and hold a kitten or adult cat against its will if it wants to get away from you; to try to restrain it will provoke an attack, so let it go!

If your own cat does scratch you, do not hit or over-scold it. Instead, hold the cat's face to the injured place and then declare, 'Look what you have done to me. What a cruel cat!' Cats do possess a strong sense of shame and very probably will not scratch you again (or at least not many times more) if you act similarly each time you are scratched.

Cat claws

One does not want cat claws to grow too long and so more dangerous. Trimming of claws is not usually necessary when a cat leads an active life which includes much time out of doors – wild cats do not have to have their claws trimmed. But cats which spend most of their time indoors may need attention to their claws.

Oil the nails with castor oil for several days before cutting to make this easier. The very tip of the nail is the only part to be cut: to cut more than just the tip will damage the claw, and its claws are very vital to the cat. Use the same type of scissors used for trimming human nails.

If one does get a deep cat scratch, then treat it with a herbal lotion that is both antiseptic and soothing for it is sometimes possible for cat scratch fever to develop. Make a strong brew of the most antiseptic of the herbs, such as sage, rosemary, geranium, yarrow, and add a few spice cloves for their soothing property. Bathe the place frequently with this brew.

If one is scratched, wash immediately with water and apply a little lemon juice. In addition to the recommended herbal treatment, one can make up a scratch dressing to be kept in a bottle. Steep well-crushed spice cloves in any light vegetable oil (not heavy olive oil), three cloves to each teaspoon of oil. The dressing can be further improved by the addition of a teaspoon of witch-hazel extract to every six teaspoons of the clove oil.

Against a really savage cat one can always protect one's hands with a pair of strong gloves, and *never* interfere with a cat and its food: that is asking to be scratched.

One must remember that the cat is a member of the tiger family and tiger claws are famed for their terrible power. The dog bites in self-protection or when attacking prey: the cat is a clawer and scratcher, so its claws are vital. Despite its small

15

size it is a valiant fighter against enemies, whether they be dogs, or humans wanting to take the animal for medical experiments or for its fur. So a cat's claws are vital.

DE-CLAWING

This makes a modern practice all the more deplorable. Modern cat owners in ever-increasing numbers are having a cruel, painful and often dangerous operation performed on their cats by veterinary surgeons, an operation known as declawing.

De-clawing is done to prevent cats from scratching their owners and for protection of upholstery and wood furniture in the home. Cats will often use such as scratching places to keep their claws in good trim unless they are carefully taught not to do so and are given special facilities for claw exercise as I will advise.

This veterinary operation of de-clawing is similar to cutting off the last joint of every finger of the human hand. Cat claws are like the last joints of human fingers. A cat with its claws removed by man becomes a defenceless creature. The enemy – attacking dogs and cats, in the frequent fights of cats – can do as they will with a de-clawed cat.

As well as in the killing of prey for their food, cats use their claws for many other purposes, such as the exercise of their leg muscles, brought into use when cats are stretching and contracting and pressing with their claws.

Cat claws are needed for their daily grooming, which is an important part of feline life. With their claws, they open up hair mats, remove skin parasites, and pull away thorny vegetation which has become attached to their limbs and bodies, vegetation such as fox-tail grass heads and burs. These can penetrate cat flesh and cause serious health problems.

When cats are climbing trees – an important activity – they need their claws to give grip to their feet. Tree-climbing for clawless cats becomes a very dangerous activity.

They also make use of their claws when eating their food, tearing up portions of flesh, rendering it small enough to enter their mouths, and holding food there while they chew at it because the cat is an animal with a small mouth and not very powerful teeth.

Fortunately, indeed very fortunately, this de-clawing operation is costly and it is also a difficult operation for vets to perform. Because it is a painful operation for cats to suffer, many veterinarians advise against de-clawing and refuse to operate. The high cost *does* deter cat owners from this modern practice.

On the other hand, unfortunately many cat owners do not realize the harm they are doing to their cats by paying for this operation to be performed on them.

The de-clawed cat, usually as a result of this operation, becomes aware of its handicapped and defenceless state and may become permanently depressed and unbalanced mentally, never again to be the happy, purring domestic cat.

I hope that very soon the removal of cat claws will be classed as cruelty to animals, and that those who perform this surgery and those who pay for it to be performed will be penalized by heavy fines. Only then is this modern trend likely to be stopped.

There is good news, at least in the Netherlands. A Dutch veterinary friend, Dr Cornelius Van Lee Wagen, from Holland, was visiting me and he told me that the de-clawing of cats has been outlawed in his country and no animal may be made defenceless. Vets are forbidden by law to do this operation, and would lose their rights to continue in the profession if found to have performed such mutilation.

Dr Van Lee Wagen also told me about another cruel modern operation, one performed mostly on dogs, but cats are included, and that is the manipulation of the vocal chords so that the animal is rendered voiceless. The purpose of this cruel operation is to protect owners against the annoyance of mewing and barking sounds.

Imagine the terror of an animal so operated on, that when it opens its mouth to communicate with owner or with other animals, no sound emerges: 'Dear God Pan! I am speechless. Never again can I speak my greetings, my needs, my pleasures, never bay to friend moon, nor give warnings to those whose home I share. God Pan! Let me die.'

SCRATCHING PLACES

Earlier in this chapter I have mentioned the provision of a small ladder for confined cats, the rungs padded and covered with coarse cloth to provide claw exercise (scratching) places.

It is also useful for indoor cats to give them one or two other special scratching places, and teach them to use such places by rubbing their claws up and down the rough surfaces and praising the cat when it uses them. Such scratching posts can be bought ready-made from well-equipped pet shops, or can be home-made using a strong piece of wood about three feet in length. Bind around the wood a piece of coarse cloth, such as sacking, or better still, pieces of carpet.

Cats like to exercise their claws on coarse material, and if it can be scented with favourite odours, such as pine, cedar, or the herb catmint, then it is perfection for the users-to-be.

RAISING KITTENS

Size of litters

My advice and teaching is not to burden the mother cat with the feeding of more than three kittens each litter, and to try to ensure that she does not have too frequent litters.

It is important to know that wild felines do not raise all the offspring to which they give birth. Instead, they make careful selection immediately the birthing is completed. With instinctive knowledge they select the strongest of the litter and put them on one side. Usually cats and dogs keep only three from every litter when living wild; the rejects they cover over with earth and leave them to die. The young of felines do not open their eyes until they are several weeks old, therefore the rejected ones do not see what is going on and soon die.

Unwanted kittens

As I have indicated, cats which litter in domestic surroundings should not keep more than three kittens, the strongest-looking being chosen by the human owner as domestic cats no longer possess the instinctive skill of selection.

The unwanted kittens should then be put down by a vet. If this is done immediately after the birth the kittens know no pain. If veterinary help is not readily available, then home destruction is necessary. *Never* drown new-born kittens or puppies. In the womb they are in watery protection, so water is their element and, put into water, they would not die speedily. Only, if absolutely necessary, use ether. The kitten is put into a plastic bag and a pad of cotton wool, soaked in ether, is applied to its face. Death is speedy and painless: the kitten merely goes to sleep.

In most countries ether can be obtained only on a prescription, to prevent its misuse. Therefore be prepared and obtain a permit from your doctor or vet having explained for what purpose the ether is required.

I have seen several times the terrible cruelty perpetrated by humans on litters of kittens and puppies. Fully alive, they have been tied up in bags and put into street refuse bins.

Those humans responsible for such crimes should themselves be put into prison!

Training of kittens

As feline urine and excreta have a very unpleasant odour, which is difficult to clean from floors, mats and carpets in the home, cats must be taught clean habits from early kittenhood, trained carefully and thoroughly. Whereas the bitch trains her whelps in house or kennel cleanliness at a very early age, the she-cat is often uncaring in this respect and allows her kittens to urinate and excrete wherever they care to do so.

The human cat-owner has to take on this training task.

Litter-trays need to be used at first (or used always if the cat is house-confined). I recommend the addition of some ash from wood fires, or charcoal dust if the former is not available. Both absorb odour very effectively and also deter house flies.

Quite apart from use in litter, I advise wood ash for another purpose, to be provided in boxes for the kittens to eat. These boxes should be raised quite high so that the kittens do not think they are litter-trays. Clean earth is equally good and necessary and by 'clean' I mean pollution free, uncontaminated by vehicle fumes, pesticides and herbicides. Clean wood ash and earth are eaten by kittens and pups with avidity, to remove worms and to supply minerals and trace elements. (Human children are also known to eat earth for similar reasons.) I have also often seen fox-cubs feasting on earth: they seem to prefer the finely-sifted earth from molehills, which is also good earth for kittens and puppies.

OBEDIENCE

Kittens and adult cats being trained in obedience, learning to follow the human commands of 'No!' and 'You must not do *that*!' (as with the dog) need to be rewarded for obedience by the giving of suitable 'titbits'. In the case of cats, such things as small squares of butter (not harmful margarine): all cats love butter. Or anything fishy out of a tin, and I do not mean tinned foods sold specifically for felines, but fish foods for human use such as sardines, salmon or anchovies. A praising human voice, human hand caresses and good things to eat are the best way to reward cats for being obedient.

Removing kittens from their mother

In the raising of cats, something must be said about the removal of kittens from the mother when the time comes for them to go to new homes. Make sure they are *good* homes and also ensure that they are not likely ever to end up as tortured *laboratory* cats.

First, the kittens should not leave their mother all on the same day: that is heartbreak for her. Remove them over a week or so, leaving one with her for longer to draw off her breast milk and to comfort her in the loss of the others. In the wild, the young stay with their mother long after weaning.

One must also consider the heartbreak of the kitten, going away from the warmth and security of its family life. Before the kittens are due to leave their mother, many pieces of cloth (cotton, not nylon) should be placed where they sleep with their mother. Those pieces of cloth will soon acquire the odours of mother and kittens, and the kitten, if given a piece of such cloth with the family scent strongly on it, will be comforted quite effectively in its new home. The cloths should have been in use in the family nest for at least one week to get well scented.

Details of diet need to go along with every kitten so that there will not be a further upset of diet change, as well as of loneliness in the new home. The kitten needs to continue on its sensible and healthy nature diet.

An old-fashioned way to help a kitten to settle well into a new home and not run away and be lost in its early days is, I think, charming.

The help is to butter its paws, all four of them, and to butter them well! By the time the kitten has licked the butter off its paws it has become fairly familiar with its new surroundings; and if the buttering of paws is repeated for several following days, a contented, new-home kitten is in place.

Naming a kitten

Give a new kitten its name immediately. The calling of that chosen word, its name, by its new owner, is also comforting. (Gypsies vow it is unlucky for animals of all kinds not to be named as soon as they are owned by a human family.) In Chapter 5 of this book I give cat names in quantity, for they are intriguing.

SURVIVAL OF CATS

In this chapter on the raising of cats, mention must be made of the cat's legendary nine lives for there seems to be much truth in this reputation, which applies only to cats, not to any other animal and not to man.

The general make-up of the cat may be partly responsible for its amazing survival when death seems positive. For instance, despite the smallness of its head, the cat has an extremely quick and keen brain, enabling it to act quickly and positively in dangerous situations.

Remembering all this, do not decide too hastily to have a badly injured cat 'killed to end its misery'. For that very cat may yet make use of one of its blessed nine chances of recovery. Therefore give every cat the chance to survive in

RAISING THE DOMESTIC CAT

situations when survival would not be possible for any other species of animal. I have witnessed, or heard of, many cases of remarkable recovery from death made by sick or injured cats, or cats buried beneath collapsed buildings in wars or earthquakes. Here are two typical examples.

Mexico. The cat of my friend, Professor Edmond Bordeaux Szekely, was bitten in a front leg by a rattlesnake of a very dangerous type, a bite that was usually fatal. This cat, Arriman, refused all human help, clawing himself away from his frantic owner who loved the cat deeply. Arriman crawled away to a nearby river and waded deep into the water. And there he remained for three days, thigh deep, drinking the river water and eating a coarse floating grass for medicine. He then emerged from the river, fully recovered. I witnessed this case from its beginning to its happy end.

Greece. Another nine lives example! In a recent earthquake in Kalamata in the Peloponnese, wherein there was much loss of life, human and animal, mostly from collapsed buildings, the mewing of a cat was heard quite loudly from a small house which was a total ruin.

The earthquake had been ten days before. No human or animal survivors were expected.

A rescue team pulled away much of the rubble and to the surprise of everyone there emerged two cats, an elderly woman and many hens, in that order. (Poultry is not unusual in primitive houses in Greece.) That company of human, fur and feather had survived those ten days with almost no air and only a small amount of water. None was injured but all were thirsty and hungry. Two cats with their nine lives had been there to give safety in that dangerous situation. The cat cries had brought help just in time.

And helpfully, just as I am writing this part of my cats book, there has come on my radio an account of another remarkable cat survival. On the BBC World Service it was told that a cat, Felix by name, being sent to England, was lost in the cargo hold of a Jumbo jet plane. The cat was in the hold for fourteen days during which time he had made many flights to far countries. Possibly he had access to a little water, but no food. When found, he was still in good health. This further upholds what I have written about fasting sick cats. Not to worry, for cats can remain alive very long without food.

It seems that Felix was having his last fling before he had to undergo the painful confinement of modern quarantine law. I hope his two weeks in the Jumbo jet were deducted from the six months of quarantine prison!

HEALTH HAZARDS

There are new dangers in life today for our pet cats, dogs and birds, if confined within town apartments, and those are pollution from the teeming motor traffic and fumes from oil and gas heaters entering through windows. These can be controlled a little by careful ventilation.

Then there is also the tobacco hazard from humans smoking cigarettes and pipes. The animals sharing the apartments of smokers are made unwilling inhalers of the poison fumes. (Of domestic pets, caged birds are the worst sufferers from tobacco smoke.) Windows should always be opened when humans are smoking. Better the exhaust fumes from motors than the nicotine smoke.

There are also health dangers from television sets, particularly colours sets, and from modern microwave ovens. They all emit radiations which are harmful to health so keep all pets from going too close to them.

NATURAL LIFE FOR CATS

Finally, the worst problem with which the modern cat (and other domestic pets and larger animals, especially farm ones that are confined for intensive farming) has to cope is monotony in its life, often total boredom.

The natural life of animals, especially the wild ones, is very active and filled with interest, such as the hunting of food, courtship, raising of young ones, also the bracing contact with the elements, far travel (for the meat-eating animals like to move continually to new territories in order to find sufficient prey for their needs). This constant movement prevents the land from becoming fouled from over-use and over-concentration of urine and faeces, which are both destructive to the earth, unlike the droppings from vegetarian animals, which are beneficial.

It is deeply painful to think about the imprisoned existence of the millions of farm animals which today are subjected to what is called 'intensive farming' (to me, devil's farming). They are deprived of all normal exercise and of their natural foods, and mostly deprived of the right of all creatures to have progeny. This last cruel ban is also often the lot of modern home animals, the cat and dog.

This is all defiance of God's care and decree for his animals when He arranged their safe travel in his miraculous Ark, and they were put there in pairs so that they could 'multiply', and their special food needs were provided. Everyone should read George Orwell's book, *Animal Farm*: it is prophetic.

Important! When a pet animal has to be confined indoors for most of every day, with the resultant acute boredom, is it not a good idea to consider keeping a pair of animals instead of a solitary one? It sends a lasting ray of happiness into an animal's life if it is no longer compelled to be alone, to be able to converse and play with a fellow creature. The devotion that animals show to one another does not interfere at all with the different devotion they have for their owners, which is often deeper.

It is popular in Great Britain, particularly in London and other urban areas, for owners to keep two cats, but there seem to be no set rules about choosing the pairings – older and younger cat, or two from the same litter, or other combinations. Indeed I know of one instance of two kittens taken from the same litter who from the beginning have acted independently of each other: they come and go at different times and one sticks firmly to the husband, the other to the wife, although the wife feeds both of the cats! The answer is that cats are like people; each one is an individual with individual preferences.

Wild and feral cats

In former times (probably best defined as *before* the age of the motor vehicle), the domestic cat when a city-dweller was never totally confined indoors.

Mankind was kinder then, less spiteful and selfish towards creatures of all kinds, and the free-moving cat was part of city life. Cats prowled the streets and leapt around on roof-tops where they serenaded the moon. Just as the canines bay at the moon, above all the full moon, cats *scream* at the moon in feline ecstasy.

Semi-wild cats, which used to be called alley cats, free from any attachment to humans, streaked around in the streets and hunted in ruins and on the city refuse places, keeping down the rats and mice, which are a bad and dangerous part of every city without exception. Today, the alley cat is a rarity, although there are some groups of feral cats in London, notably Camden Town, as was shown in an interesting programme on British television. But semi- and truly wild cats are still to be found in country places, and I have often met with them and always admired them for their supple bodies and brilliant eyes. The wild cats in Scotland, for instance, can be really fierce.

On Greek islands it is not rare to meet with true wild cats of the lonely places, often cave-dwellers. Savage, cruel-clawed creatures, able to rear their litters of kittens in excellent health, those cat families subsist entirely on food taken from sea-coast pools and from the inland tree-groves.

It was in Holland that I had closest contact with two wild cats, though I felt they were domestic cats turned wild, for they were mild of character and did not possess the menacing ferocity of the true wild cat such as I met in Israel and North Africa. But the Dutch cats were the most beautiful. Woodlands bordering the moorlands of Drenthe were their dwelling place, but very heavy snow brought them to the farm where I was living, and they took cereals from the feed-bins (for cats, like dogs and foxes, will eat cereals and digest them well when flesh is not available). That pair of cats, however, soon found and ate small animal prey when people were not around, for very soon after they were first seen the snow began to be littered with scraps of fur and with feathers.

What beautiful, fiery-eyed cats were those of Drenthe! With what suppleness and rhythm they moved, so wild! I longed to photograph them, but at the slightest sound of human footsteps on the snow they fled out of sight.

EXERCISE FOR TOWN CATS

The boredom of confined city cats can be alleviated by training them to take walks on long, light leashes such as are sold in pet shops for Siamese cats, which are almost doglike in the way they adapt to leash exercise. It is most difficult to train other species of cat to this form of exercise, but it can be done. I have done it and so have many other people as advised by me in my book, *The Complete Herbal Handbook for the Dog and Cat* (Faber and Faber), which managed to get itself translated into four languages.

It is necessary to *train* cats to accept anything unusual to their natures, such as leash-walking or being bathed, necessary to train from kitten age, then success is sure.

Dogs are happy leash-walkers; in fact they demand their daily walks from their owners and they may sulk and become destructive in the home if denied this pleasure. Nose to ground, the dog on walks reads the newspapers of the streets, reads not by sight but by scent. The cat also does its walks-reading, but its reading is not like that of the dog.

On leash-walks cats do not sniff the ground, they carry their heads high and take their scenting from the air and they use their eyes sharply. It is as well to remember that cats on leashes are apt to get entangled, so the leash should be held short.

When walking-out cats in cities one must be aware of danger from stray dogs who are off leash. Do not take any risks: lift up the leashed cat immediately any unleashed dog is sighted. If savage dogs are known to be around in one's walking area, then carry a small bag of black pepper and if any dog leaps at the cat in one's arms, fling some of the pepper at the nose of the attacker: it will be subdued at once, but keep the pepper away from the villain's eyes. A dog-chain with which to hit an attacking dog is also helpful.

Cats on leashes are not only to be seen in towns. I well recall a Spanish gypsy woman, in a woodland grove beyond Malaga, Andalucia. She was of the true nomad type but she used no horse, mule or donkey; she was a foot-traveller and she took her cats on her endless journeyings as well as her dogs. I took a photograph of her (and this has been published

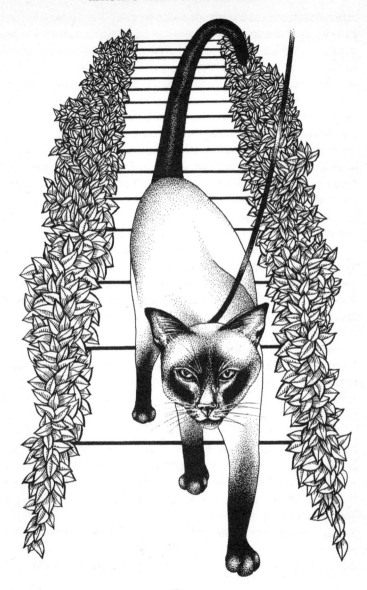

in several European journals) with her two big tabby cats and two dogs of terrier type. The dogs ran free, but the two cats were on leashes and walked, well trained, at their owner's side.

Dogs and cats all wore jingling bells, which made a pretty sound. Over one of the gypsy's arms was a large basket which, she told me, was for her cats; she lifted them up into the basket when they showed any sign of foot-tiredness. Her only other 'luggage' was a back-pack in which she kept some loaves of bread and pieces of cheese, food for her animals and herself. They all looked in good health, therefore I expect she supplemented bread and cheese with other foods from the woods and fields, which her animals helped her to find.

Many country cats will voluntarily accompany their owners on their walks, off leash of course, prancing around and thoroughly enjoying themselves. Cats are also well known for making incredible journeys back to homes which they loved when, for some reason or other, they were removed from there. Journeys back to 'the home hearth' of a hundred miles or so are known to have happened. Sometimes those 'removed' cats are months away, and then, there they are, back by their former familiar place, footsore, thin, but determined and happy.

Entertainment for cats

Not only do dogs love to travel with their owners in cars (with a few exceptions who suffer from car nerves) but most cats enjoy such travel, so to reduce daily boredom for animals make a habit of taking the family cat, possibly with the dog too, for frequent car rides.

Put a collar and leash on the cat, a collar bell and a clearly-written name and address label in case the cat jumps from the car and gets lost. If windows are not opened too wide there should be no danger in that respect. Hear how the cat purrs when the collar and leash are brought out for the car ride into places where the air is fresh and sweet from fields and trees.

Cat dens

Having stressed the importance of exercise and entertainment for health and happiness, I now turn to the importance for confined cats of their own special 'den' (their tiger lair). That true cat-lover, the novelist Doris Lessing, says of cats, 'A cat needs a *place* as much as it needs a person to make its own.'

Preferably the cat den should be in the quietest part of the human home. All domestic cats need their own place where they can go and rest when inclined and also sleep. The quietness of such a place is stressed because the supersensitive ears of the cat suffer when subjected to constant noise from human voices or, yet worse, radio or television turned to high volume of sound.

The den should be in a dimly-lit place for true comfort, and for the cat's bed a wooden box is best, holding a cushion of cotton cloth filled with cotton padding. If cedar-wood shavings or chips, or likewise of pine trees, can be obtained and also put into the cat's bed-cushion, this will keep the cat very contented as it loves the scent of both. The cat has another favoured scent, that of the herb *Nepeta* (*Nepeta cataria*, Labiatae) called catmint or catnip. If some catmint in dried form could be put into the cat's bed, what joy!

No nylon or woollen bedding should be used: the former is unhealthy, the latter breeds skin vermin such as fleas and lice. A basket is often used for a cat bed and does look more attractive than a wooden box, but a basket is a sure breeding-place for fleas and other pests and should not be used. A wooden box can be kept clean with ease and can be replaced by a new one occasionally, not being as expensive as a basket.

Fleas

The cat flea must be prevented from establishing itself in the home because, once it has made its place in house furnishings and carpets, it is very difficult to eradicate because of its smallness (and its cunning).

The cat flea is small and black, a true menace, and a persistent biter of humans, compared with the bigger, brown, dog flea which is much easier to catch. Fleas are dealt with more fully in Chapter 4.

Bathing

It is a small jump from fleas to baths for cats, a very vexed matter. Although cats will willingly wade into sea pools and streams to catch fish, many of them dislike being bathed and will scratch in order to escape the bathing.

Therefore teach bathing in early kittenhood, even if it is not needed then. Make mock baths of shallow water depth and make the bath more secure for the kitten by placing a towel, weighted down, at the bottom of the bath to prevent slipping feet. Use warm water, and praise and pat the kitten, making the bathing a pleasing experience instead of a frightening one.

3

Nature Diet for Cats

Vegetarian foods, Size of feeds, Cats and birds, Fresh foods, Herbs, Diet for health, Flesh foods, Fish, Bones, Milk, Cheese, Cereals, Other foods for cats, Oil for cats, 'Pet foods', Raw foods, Legumes, Natural Rearing Diets, NR Diet for kittens, Weaning, NR Diet for adult cats

The character of the cat is shown in its food preferences. By character the cat is strong, self-willed and frugal and likes its foods in small amounts only, fresh and natural. If one wants to own a healthy and contented cat its feeding inclinations must be kept in mind.

For example, the house dog will accept, and enjoy, meat that has turned 'gamey', that is high-smelling from long keeping, and it will even eat maggoty flesh if it finds such. A cat, however, will refuse all flesh which is not fresh.

Vegetarian foods

All the felines and carnivores need grains and vegetable foods in addition to flesh. They obtain such vegetarian foods in semi-digested form when devouring the stomachs and intestines of prey which they have killed. It is notable that on making a 'kill' they first rip open the abdomen and devour the contents of the stomach and intestinal tract.

In a BBC (Britain) series on zoos of the world, it was stated that the keeper of the 'big cats' at Munich Zoo, West Germany, had great success with them. He credited that success to his method of feeding them quantities of vegetable-filled stomach and intestines from slaughterhouses, given raw.

It is known that the carnivore foxes of Europe and elsewhere, deprived of their usual diet of rabbits, become largely vegetarian, feeding on young cereals and on vegetables and fruits, and keep in excellent health.

Modern foxes in their own way paid back the farmer for his cruel destruction of the rabbit population (by deliberate spreading of a killer rabbit virus) by eating up the foods for which man killed the rabbits for taking from his lands in the first place!

Cats and dogs all enjoy fresh hedgerow berries, grapes, nuts, and many sorts of vegetable. In the Bible it is mentioned that the foxes 'spoil the tender vines', and I have seen great destruction in the melon fields of the Middle East, caused by jackals feeding on the melons. Cats will also bite with enjoyment into ripe melons and they have a passion for ripe cucumbers.

All animals enjoy corn cobs when the kernels within them are tender, sweet and milky. Indeed, corn, a very important food, can be given in flaked (crushed) form, or as corn puffs, which are now a popular commercial food in many countries. Nuts of all kinds when soft and fresh are also popular with all animals.

When choosing a nature diet for one's cat remember, therefore, not to feed flesh foods only and absolutely *avoid* giving canned cat foods, or meat or fish.

If one consistently feeds a nature diet to one's cat or cats, the following chapter on ailments of the cat will not have to be read at all: it will never be used!

Size of feeds

Remember, too, that the cat has a small stomach capacity and cannot manage on the one or two meals a day of the dog. The cat needs at least three small meals daily if it is a domestic cat and not free to roam the fields and forage for itself.

When it is free to roam it is a great provider. The American author and naturalist, Svevo Brooks, told me about a young female house cat, who formerly had lived well on left-overs from the farm table with milk and raw eggs also given. She gave birth to many kittens in a nearby stable and needed far more food than that fed to her from the house table.

This cat, although only young, became a 'mighty hunter'. Daily she could be seen returning to the stable carrying home such fare as mice, young rabbits, squirrels, lizards and (unfortunately) birds. When her kittens had grown and homes had been found for them, she no longer hunted her own food but returned to the scraps from the home table: necessity had turned her into a hunter for the time being and feline inherited intelligence had made her a success.

Cats and birds

An aside about cats as bird-killers: they should be discouraged from killing birds, which are so important to our world as eaters of insects and distributors of seeds as well as for the delight of their singing.

Cats should be scolded and told they are 'bad' each time they bring home a bird. The bird should be *snatched* from them and some other well-liked food given to them instead of the bird. A confirmed, addicted bird-killer, and I have had them in my gardens from time to time, should be fitted with a collar and bell, a bell loud enough to alert the birds. Take care that the collar fits well to the neck so it cannot be caught up on twigs of trees and bushes, on fencing and other projections, and thus cost the cat its life instead of the birds being protected! For such protection, a collar with breaks easily should be used.

Here also is the place for another aside, this one about mice and birds which cats seem to like to bring home with them, even when they have no kittens to feed, as if they want to show off their hunting skills to their owners.

The cat upsets its human owner by the seemingly wilfully cruel treatment which it metes out to the prey it has caught. Cats bring home their prey alive, mostly, and then they claw at it and toss it with their paws, free their victim, then pounce and recapture. The true fact is that this is not torture, but they are softening up their prey internally to make them easier for eating. Indeed, when their victims are pulped internally, cats will often swallow them whole.

The reason for this seems to be that the cat knows that once the flesh is torn and the smell of blood is around, this smell may attract some other larger creature who may swoop down and deprive the cat of its prey. That also is the reason why the cat likes to bring home what it has captured; it does so for its own good and not to impress or please it owners, for, once home, it feels safer from attack from other animals who may steal what it has caught. It may have been caught after much care and difficulty as small animals become increasingly scarce, killed off by man's foolish and selfish use of pesticides and herbicides over the countryside which once, a long time ago, was all blossoming and safe.

FRESH FOODS

It is notable that foods fresh from the field are far more acceptable to animals than are those raised on commercial farms; especially unpopular are the meat foods raised by the intensive (devilish) method.

Here is an interesting note concerning the difference between flesh from wild creatures and from those raised in intensive places, and it concerns snakes. A snake-keeper and raiser, whom I met recently in Scotland, told me that field-caught rats and mice fed to his snakes (large types such as boas and pythons) are eaten up immediately, whereas those purchased from sources raising rodents for supplies to such places as zoos, rodents which are confined and have no access to fresh field foods but are fed concentrated pellets which are lifeless and heavy with chemical preservatives, remain untouched for days until hunger provokes the eating of them. Snakes also like to eat live food, so the dead food has to be moved with a stick to make pretence that it is living!

The basic law for nature diet for our cats, therefore, should be food as fresh as possible and no foods out of commercial cans except occasionally some of the (not for pets) fish or cereal foods, safe from heavy chemical preservation, because they are sold *for human use*. If one's cats can go out into the countryside and obtain their own food, so much the better!

Herbs

Part of a nature diet is the provision of health herbs. If the cat has not access to such in home garden or in fields beyond the garden, then they should be provided in pots so that the cats can pull and chew at them. The cat is not quite the super-skilled self-herbalist as are the dog and fox, but is efficient none the less.

The most important feline herbs to provide in pots are garlic (cats pull and chew at the leaves), borage (cats also like the leaves of this plant), couch grass, maidenhair fern, and the cats' favourite herb, catmint (also called catnip). Cats not

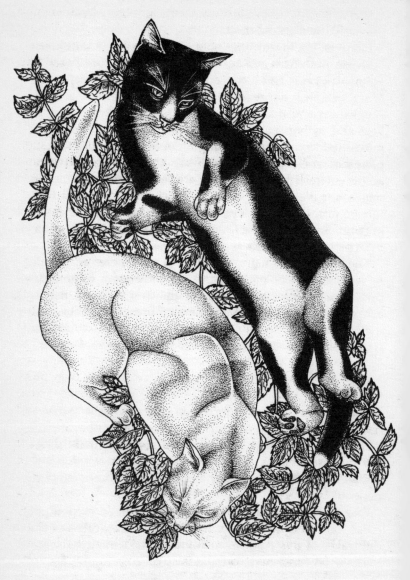

only chew up this mint-type herb, if it is in large enough quantity and growing in the earth, not in pots, they love to roll in catmint. This 'rolling-in-the-mint' of cats is not purely for joy and good scent, the herb is a skin vermin deterrent and also a herb tonic.

Diet for health

My diet for the natural feeding of kittens and adult cats (and I have a similar and not very different diet for puppies and adult dogs) is known as Natural Rearing, and has been in use for more than fifty years, so it has been very well tested. Indeed, NR animals are in demand world wide because of their well-known excellent health and the good temperaments which are typical of healthy animals with a strong and well-balanced nervous system.

In supplying diets it is not possible ever to give exact amounts. Cat-owners must watch their kittens and adult cats to see if they seem well satisfied and well nourished on the amounts suggested. If the cat grows over-thin, then amounts of food should be increased. The quantity of food needed to nourish a growing or fully-grown cat differs with many factors: breed of cat (mongrels usually need more than purebred cats), temperament, amount of exercise being taken, climate (cats in hot climates eat less than those in cool or cold climates), and so on.

Kittens should be carefully watched for over-feeding. If their stomachs appear bloated, then reduce the amount of food being given.

Cats, more so than dogs, like variety in their food, and if they do not get this and are kept on a monotonous diet, they may well turn into finicky eaters, leave much of their food uneaten and consequently lose body condition and become ill. Therefore aim at variety.

To repeat myself, but I want to stress the point, the best diet for cats, indeed for all creatures, including man, is made up from freshly-gathered or killed foods, wild produce from the countryside (if not poisoned with herbicides, which take a while to show their presence), or foods organically grown and thus free from chemical fertilizers and poison sprays. Unfortunately nowadays such foods are not very plentiful and too often are very highly priced because demand generally exceeds supply. But try and feed at least *some* organic foods.

Flesh foods

Vary the kinds of flesh foods used: mutton (lamb), poultry, rabbit. Avoid the coarse flesh of beef as cats never eat such flesh. A cat, unlike a dog, could never kill cattle, and really not sheep or goats either, although they can enjoy the two latter if fed cut into small pieces and could be allowed it if it is more convenient for their owners to feed some butcher's shop meat. (In writing here of cats I do not, of course, include the large cats such as lions and tigers.)

Permission for domestic cats to eat butcher's meat does not apply to cow meat and certainly not to pork, the latter being a medium for encysted tapeworm when cats and other meat-eaters feed on such flesh; the intestines of rabbits are also the carriers of tapeworm when eaten by cats. Strictly avoid pork, including the bones. Pig flesh (except that of wild pigs) is apt to be over-fat, greasy, indigestible and generally unhealthy for cats.

When feeding meat, always feed it raw. Cooking meat kills the vitality of flesh, softens it and does in the cooking what the digestive juices of the cat should be doing in the process of digesting raw flesh. Likewise minced meat is harmful as it weakens the digestive system and encourages over-eating. Minced meat weakens the eater as it deprives the digestive juices and internal muscles of their work and prevents them from being kept exercised in the breaking-down and digestion of raw flesh, the predominant food of the felines.

Feed only a little fat. Unlike the meat from domestic animals, the meat of wild creatures – the natural diet of the cat – is lean meat always because wild animals are unlikely to become very fat. If there is much fat on bought meat, throw away the fat rather than having to pay expensive veterinary fees for treatment of ailments of liver or pancreas which result from the intake of too much fat.

Fish

Fresh fish is much liked by cats and is excellent food for them. If the fish is freshly caught by cat-owners (one seldom finds fresh-caught fish in shops) then it can be fed raw. Cats themselves are often seen catching their own fish from shallow coastal pools. They do not need such catches to be cooked and eat them up as they catch.

Fish, however, like rabbits and poultry, hardens quickly after death and becomes indigestible, so all three types of food require some light cooking to resoften the flesh. Steaming or baking are the best forms of cooking: never fry fish because frying is as bad for the health as greasy pork.

Cats like very much fish that is canned for human use and this is permissible because such fish is subject to government control and does not contain dangerous chemical preservatives which are often used without discrimination or control in canned fish products sold for pets.

All cats have a liking for canned sardines and salmon. Tuna fish was once a popular food to feed to cats, but is not now used much because tuna seem prone to take in radio-active particles. It is, therefore, a suspect food and needs to be tested before use.

Bones

Although all cats love meaty bones they are often deprived of them by their owners because of fears that they might cause choking or internal damage. Bones are vital to the health of teeth and jaws and to the entire digestive system, as well as for cats' pleasure in eating and playing with them, and also exercise for feet and claws.

Do not misuse bones. Never cook them because, once they have been cooked, many bones can break up into sharp splinters when being eaten and can cause death by internal puncture of the digestive organs. (I know of many such deaths in cats and dogs.) Poultry bones are especially apt to splinter when cooked, but the raw bony heads and legs of poultry are good and inexpensive food for cats. Beaks and claws should be cut off, and heads and legs partly shredded with a sharp knife to make them easier to eat as they are rather tough.

As a safety measure I never feed very small bones, nor much gristle, to either cats or dogs and this ban applies to small bones even when in a raw state. Bones should be fed *after*, not before meals.

Despite the fact that cats and dogs are natural carnivores, do not feed them too much meat or fish. It is logical that neither cat nor dog in the wild could kill prey daily; there would be days in the week when no kill would be made. So, remember this, and do not feed flesh more than four days a week. This also applies to fish, which is included in the flesh allowance. On other days the meals should be made up of milk products and cereals.

Milk

Cats enjoy a saucer of milk, although this needs to be introduced into their diet at weaning time. Otherwise the grown cat may refuse milk, which would be a pity because milk, if obtained from healthy animals, is such an excellent and internally soothing food, and is not expensive. Some forms of milk, such as sour milk and buttermilk, are also health remedies, which soothe the digestive organs and deter or remove worms.

Some cats not healthy enough to digest raw milk may do better on yoghurt, the plain variety. Indeed, some cats seem to prefer yoghurt to fresh milk and lap it up with much enjoyment.

All types of fresh milk are permissible, but the preferred ones are goat or sheep milks. Do not heat the milk in the mistaken idea that one is killing so-called germs of disease. Heating of milk kills all its vitality and changes its properties so that, on keeping for a short time, it does not turn to a healthy sour state, but turns to a stinking, rotten state and is then harmful, far more harmful than the feared germs.

For more than half a century I've used only raw milk in my own diet and that of my children and my animals. Milk is known to be a great restorer in illness, especially when diluted with barley water and fortified with honey. The Greeks, who are mostly cat-lovers and far kinder to their cats than to their chained-up dogs, declare that for any cat ailment the one supreme medicine is fresh milk, slightly warmed. But it should be mentioned that in most parts of Greece milk is still natural and not the modern, dead 'long-life' stuff sold in cartons or plastic containers or tins.

Products of milk: butter and cheese. All cats love fresh butter but, being very rich and indigestible, it should be fed only in small amounts. The small amount necessary to butter a new kitten's paws, which I have described earlier, is permissible.

Margarine, which is not usually made from milk and is commonly made from the fat of our ill-fated whales, *should be*

43

avoided totally. It is hydrolysed fat and never fully dissolves when eaten. We all know of the 'ever-keeping' qualities of margarine: it never goes bad or sour. This property means that it lines the digestive tract when eaten and, in time, hardens the digestive system and causes true health problems.

Cheese

Soft, white cheese is excellent for cats and is a useful food on their meatless or fishless days. Hard, yellow cheese should be avoided, although cats love the taste of it. As a treat, a little yellow cheese can be given occasionally, but it should be finely grated for digestibility.

Cheese-water, poured over flaked cereals, is also an excellent cat food, and worm-expelling. This liquid is made in the pressing of cheese or in the drips from cheese being drained of its whey while it hardens. Feed cheese-water raw, uncooked.

Cereals

All cats enjoy cereals and in the wild would get them in a partly-digested state from the stomach and intestines of prey which they have killed.

The best form of cereals for cats, other than stale, wholegrain breads, is cereal in flaked form. In the flaking process the cereal grains are warmed and become sufficiently digestible to be well utilized by the cat without further cooking. Wheat is the most difficult to digest in flaked form, so I do not give wheat flakes to cats, only give wheat as wholemeal bread, either lightly buttered or softened in milk. Oats and corn are the most nourishing and barley is the most internally soothing.

44

All cats and dogs love corn and will eat it fresh off the cob when it is very young and milky. They also love tinned corn (corn and pineapple are said to be the only foods which do not lose much of their vitality or vitamins when tinned).

Cooked rice is also a good food for cats and enjoyed by them. Soak the cereal overnight to lessen the cooking time, for any form of cooking tends to spoil the food. Cats need rice to be cooked well: on no account feed rice which is hard from under-cooking.

An occasional meal of spaghetti is a treat enjoyed by cats and is quite healthful. Sprinkle it generously with finely chopped herbs and some grated hard cheese. Note that a mixture of finely-cut herbs, so important to feline health, can be given on cereals as well as flesh foods.

Other foods for cats

Lentils can be enjoyed by cats provided that they, like rice, are soaked overnight and cooked well.

Other unusual foods for cats are coconut and carrots, both in finely-grated form, for they supply minerals and vitamins and deter, even expel, worms.

All nuts can be added to cat food as a rich source of minerals, especially almonds. They need to be given finely ground. Walnuts and hazelnuts, too, could in the wild be obtained in crushed form from the intestines of prey killed by cats.

Finally eggs: all cats enjoy and benefit from raw eggs, given to them occasionally only. In the wild, cats are known to steal the eggs of wild birds. Modern thinking condemns raw egg whites, based on findings from unnatural experiments; feed eggs raw, as in the wild.

Oil for cats

Cats also need some oil to help keep their hair healthy and, in the case of long-haired cats, to help that hair to grow. Oil also helps to remove internal hair balls. I do not advise heavy olive oil. Sesame, sunflower and corn oil are best for cats. Do not risk so-called 'salad' oils as they may be of uncertain mixture and can be dangerous.

'Pet foods'

At this is a book of natural health for cats, I need not give much space to 'pet foods', sold in tins and bags (the bags usually of plastic) for cats. Almost without exception they are unnatural and therefore no friend to feline health: indeed such foods can be foe.

Fortunately in our time there has been published by Rodale Press, of Emmaus, Pa, USA, a massive book by Richard H. Pitcairn and his wife, Susan Hubble Pitcairn, which is called *Natural Health for Dogs and Cats*. In Chapter 2, entitled 'What's Really in Pet Food', the Pitcairns inform the reader of the great dangers from these modern commercial foods, which are manufactured and sold (sold well by clever commercial advertising) with little control over the types of flesh in the fish or meat foods and the chemical preservatives also used. Likewise, there is little control over the chemicals used to make the biscuit-type foods long-keeping and resistant to insect pests.

The Pitcairns warn that in almost all states in the USA pet-food makers are allowed to use what are called '4D' sources: 'Tissues from animals that are dead, dying, disabled or diseased when they arrive at the slaughterhouse.' Other pet-food ingredients include foods rejected by the USDA for human consumption, such as mouldy grains or rancid animal fats.

The authors tell that blood-soaked sawdust from slaughter-house floors, such as blood soaked in adrenalin acid from the intense terror of the animals immediately before and during slaughter, is commonly purchased by makers of pet foods to mix into their foods.

Who is to see? Who is to know that this is being done? High profits only are the reason behind the manufacture of many pet foods. The obvious conclusion to all this is simply, as in former times when there was no pet-food industry, to make your own pet foods. Feed the wholesome and beneficial things, fresh fish and meat, fresh cereals and vegetables such as I have described in this chapter.

Another quote from the Pitcairns' important book supports this chapter of mine:

Another missing ingredient is Life. All processed pet foods – whether sold in cans, bags or frozen packages, in either giant supermarkets or local health stores – are missing something which seems to me to be one of the most important 'nutrients' of all. The key ingredient is something scientists have practically ignored. But when it's there you and I can know and feel it. It is a quality found only in freshly grown uncooked whole foods. It's life energy.

Raw foods

We all know that raw foods contain more vitamins, minerals and general vitality than cooked foods, and that raw foods prevent over-eating – one can eat twice the amount of food once it has been cooked (compare, for example, a raw cabbage with a cooked one). And who could plant a field with cooked or frozen grains and expect to reap a harvest? None: for the cooked or frozen grains would be dead and would not grow.

Therefore, I repeat, for the health's sake of your cats, *feed* them naturally.

Now I want to advise on the foods which are the most life-giving, yes, life-giving, and I urge new owners to give their cats such foods as my own animals have had daily for many generations.

Apart from raw meat and fish and dairy products, most important are leafy greens from the garden or the wild or the greengrocer. Although I give here just a short list, any leafy greens except the bitter plants or the few which are poisonous, can be used.

Here are the ones I give to my cats and dogs (and to my human family): parsley, celery, mint, the sprouting leaves from onions, garlic and chives, all the cresses, nasturtium leaves, and the wild greens: sorrel, plantain, cleavers (goosegrass), dandelion (all the many varieties), chickweed, clovers (also all varieties), land and water cresses, and nettles (which need very light cooking). A suggested daily ration is a heaped teaspoon.

Because cats have difficulty in digesting raw greens, whereas in nature they would get them crushed from the intestines of their prey, the owner should cut up the greens very fine with a pair of sharp scissors or a parsley mill. This provision of daily leaves is the most time-consuming in the preparation of a nature diet, but it is very important for health. I never miss out on it and I advise those who purchase animals of my rearing not to fail in this provision of daily greens.

Cats and dogs will eat many of the listed green foods for themselves. Mine help themselves to cereals when young and green, young onion and garlic leaves, cleavers, clovers and cresses. But to make sure that they do get sufficiency of greens, provide them finely cut yourself, do not rely on the cat's inclinations.

The other vital health food for cats is sprouted grains, which can be prepared in a jar with a perforated lid. Inside the jar place a moist piece of cotton or flannel cloth (not nylon) and on that put the grains. Keep the jar in a cool place

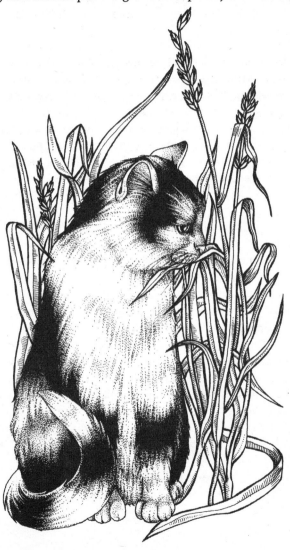

and rinse the grains twice daily to prevent the formation of mould. Any cereal grains may be used; my preferred ones are barley and maize (Indian corn). Always remember to give sprouted grains well crushed.

Legumes

This brings me to the mention of legume foods, which can also be sprouted (particularly beans and peas). Felines and carnivores love legumes, especially peas, and they do well on them and get a supply of nitrates from the legume plant family. Peas, beans and other legumes need to be fed lightly cooked, or can be fed from cans (canned baked beans for an occasional treat). Peas, beans and corn are the *only* canned foods I ever feed to my animals.

NATURAL REARING DIETS

Similar diets to those for kittens and cats have been in use for my Afghan hounds (the Turkuman Afghans) for half a century and have given me hounds known for beauty, brains and great health. Cats have a similar diet to dogs but are fed smaller quantities of food and they get more frequent meals as their digestive organs are smaller; cats get more fish and do not have beef. Puppies are more greedy feeders than kittens, so kittens need to be taught in their early days to accept milk other than that of their mother and not to reject minced raw green leafy food.

NR Diet for kittens

Kittens should be fed in individual dishes to prevent indigestion from over-quick eating from a shared dish. They should be kept on milk only until nearly four weeks. But, after three weeks of age, they can be offered extra milk to lessen the strain on their mother.

At a very early age, their second week, kittens should be offered sips of water. Dip their faces in a shallow saucer of tepid water and give praise when the kitten drinks a little. This, further, saves the mother-cat's milk from over-demand. In the wild, kittens and pups lick at dew-wet plants and drink from rain puddles.

Begin weaning kittens on warm milk fortified with flaked barley or gruel. Gruel for kittens and pups can be purchased ready-mixed, or can be made at home from: two tablespoons of flaked barley and one tablespoon each of slippery-elm flour, arrowroot flour, and one teaspoon of powdered dill seed. For each kitten take one teaspoon of this mixture and make into a paste with one teaspoon of pure honey, then stir in slowly one teaspoon of warm water (not too hot so that it destroys the vitality of the honey). Then stir in two dessertspoons of warm milk. The barley flour is more digestible if made from barley flakes. The milk used should preferably be fresh, not heated for pasteurization (which kills the goodness of the milk), nor should it be long-life milk, nor from tins.

WEANING

8 am	Gruel with milk
12 noon	Give flaked barley in milk
4 pm	Repeat 12 noon meal
8 pm	Repeat 8 am meal.

If the kittens look thin, they may need an extra feed of milk and honey at 10 pm.

One day a week feed smaller amounts of food and less frequently, so that the kittens can rest their digestive systems.

After six weeks of age (or earlier if the kittens seem to need this) feed more solid and adult foods. Confine milk and cereal feeds to 8 am and 12 noon.

Now, at 4 pm and 8 pm feed several teaspoons of cooked fish or raw meat, both fish and meat finely cut, the meat scraped with a knife, *not* minced. Add a pinch of powdered seaweed and a small teaspoon of green leafy things, finely cut, such as I have already listed in this chapter.

If the kittens are hungry they may need a repeat meal of cereal with milk.

During weaning introduce them to meaty bones, chicken legs, etc., prepared so that they can utilize them.

AFTER WEANING TO FOUR MONTHS

8 am   As much of the usual 8 am feed of milk with gruel and flaked cereals as the kitten will eat.

12 noon Omit gruel from milk and add a variety of flaked cereals in addition to barley, maize, rye, oats, but *not* wheat. Add a few drops of oil, preferably sesame, corn or sunflower, but not olive or mixed vegetable oil. Rapeseed oil is, however, permitted. Beaten raw egg can be given on some days, also cottage cheese and other soft white cheese, or buttermilk. Other healthful additions: desiccated coconut (for its rare albumen content), almonds (finely ground as flour) – only a teaspoon of each. Also grated raw carrot.

4 pm   A flesh meal of rabbit, poultry or fish, the flesh finely shredded (never minced – the mincing machine does the work which should be done by the digestive organs of the cat). Include the bones; flesh without bones is not natural. Always feed meat raw. Only rabbit, poultry and fish, unless fed immediately after being killed, before it hardens in death, may have to be lightly cooked. Give only a

small amount of fat because fat is found only in farm-raised, non-wild animals. A health hazard when feeding fat is that the body, in self-defence, isolates in its fat harmful, intaken pesticides, pollutants, hormones and other modern nonsense. Add a small teaspoon of raw bran for extra fibre because butcher's meat lacks the skin with hair or feathers which carnivores eat with the flesh. Add a sprinkle of finely-minced raw greens (already mentioned and of great importance).

8 pm   Repeat the 4 pm meal.

Note: Every kitten, from weaning onwards, should rest and cleanse its organs of digestion by having little food on one day in every week, and, on one day in every month, a fast on merely water fortified with a little honey.

Do not prevent kittens from eating such as clean earth, sand, small stones, wood-ash and charcoal, also excreta from grass-eating animals such as sheep, goats and cows. It is natural for carnivores to get vegetable food in this form.

Vinegar: When kittens get stiff-limbed and arthriticky (also adult cats), add to the drinking water a teaspoon of apple or wine vinegar (no other kind) five days a week.

Water: Provide fresh drinking water day and night. Pay attention to the quality of the water. The fluid content of all bodies is high and health depends on good water. Do not use plastic dishes; use earthenware or enamel (cracked enamel is dangerous). Change the water in the dish daily.

NR Diet for adult cats

Follow the same diet as given for older kittens, but, of course, increasing the amounts of the foods and reducing the meals to three daily.

Because cats are smaller eaters than dogs, they need more

frequent meals than the one or two needed by dogs. Those three meals already suggested should include a main meal of flesh foods, as described for kittens, a meal of milk-soaked cereals and additions such as white cheese, grated nuts and others. All foods should be given in larger amounts than described for kittens and the provision of raw bones is important.

In conclusion to this chapter on natural diet for cats, I emphasize again the importance of a well-balanced diet of fresh, whole foods, mostly fed in their raw, natural form. In modern times, the feeding of the domestic cat has cruelly and selfishly changed into a mere purchase of packeted and canned 'pet foods', which take only a few minutes to open and place in the usual plastic dish for the cat.

Daily ill-health is fed in this lazy way to the domestic cat (and likewise to the domestic dog). Often such feeding is out of ignorance, the harm being done is not realized. One does as everyone else (or almost everyone else). But there is presentday a great popular outcry against the use of so-called 'junk' foods for humans. People have become aware of the harm done to health by the eating of foods grown by chemical non-organic methods, with poisonous chemicals sprayed externally and filled internally with harmful chemicals, such food treatments being only for the convenience and ease of the growers and manufacturers. *Now* is the time to apply this ban on 'junk' foods to our cats and dogs.

For health's sake, feed a nature diet! And so check the ever-increasing ailments harming our dogs and cats, who are almost entirely dependent on their owners for their health.

4

Herbal Remedies

Gathering of herbs, Drying herbs, To make herbal brews and pills, Dosing of cats and kittens, Signs of illness, Internal cleansing, External ailments caused by insects and parasites, External ailments: other skin troubles, Ailments of the digestive system, Worms, Other common ailments, Experiments on animals

Herbs are the natural (and chosen) medicine for cats – indeed for all animals. When cats have free access to the countryside they mostly can find their own remedies to cure their ailments. However if they are house- or apartment-confined, then their owners must provide the various herbs needed for treatment of disease.

For those people interested in healing their own cats, they can obtain a copy of my book *The Illustrated Herbal Handbook for Everyone*, which contains nearly one hundred excellent, and clear, drawings of herbs by the well-known botanical artist Heather Wood. This book is now available as an inexpensive paperback in English, and in German, its title as above.

In this cat book, I have confined ailments to the really common ones. New feline ailments are ever developing and to list them all would require an over-long book out-priced far beyond purchase by the majority of cat-owners.

As I have already stated in my previous chapter, if a nature diet is consistently followed, ailments of the domestic cat will be very few, merely the common ones of the felines, distemper, mange, worms of various kinds, and skin parasites: nothing more. When a cat injures its limbs or suffers from deep cuts caused by accidents, it fasts from food and seeks out and eats medicinal herbs: and generally it is cured.

Fasting is a very important part of herbal medicine, and is followed by all creatures, by instinct, unless they are food-coaxed or force-fed by their human owners. During fasting, medicinal herbs are more effectively utilized by the animal (or likewise by the human).

Gathering of herbs

It is best (and cheapest) if cat-owners can gather their own herbs fresh from their gardens or the countryside. Gathering from the countryside is no longer so easy in present times. Dangerous chemical pesticides and herbicides are allowed to be scattered over the lands of the so-called 'developed' countries, and in some countries, the United Kingdom in particular, the law forbids the picking of certain wild plants. In the UK, too, it is illegal to uproot *any* wild plant. A list of protected species can be obtained from the Department of the Environment, Tollgate House, Houlton Street, Bristol, BS2 9DJ.

Therefore, when gathering herbs outside the control of one's own garden, make sure that it is not against the law and that the plants have not been contaminated (or poisoned) by chemical spraying, which it is not always easy to detect. For example, herbicides often take a day or more to kill those plants which have been sprayed and meanwhile may be gathered by unsuspecting people, or eaten by wild creatures. Therefore take great care when gathering herbs for yourselves or for your domestic animals.

Herbs can also be obtained in dried form from herbal shops

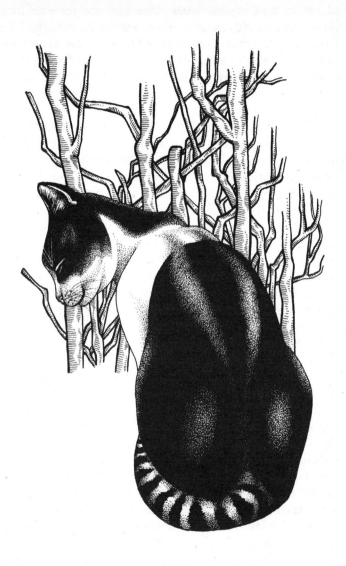

and health food stores. Make sure they are no more than twelve months old, as after that time herbs lose their full medicinal properties, especially when they are of the aromatic kind. In fact, stale herbs are worthless for medicinal purposes. When drying your own herbs, give the unused ones, when they are over a year old, to your garden or house plants as tonic compost.

Medicinal and culinary herbs should be gathered when in full leaf or in full flower. The summer solstice and the time of Saint John, June 22, are the peak times for herb-gathering. The best gathering time is around or just before midday. Do not gather herbs when their leaves are turning yellow, or when flowers are fading in colour, or when they are wet from rain or dew, or even frost. Damp herbs will not dry well and will probably turn mouldy.

DRYING HERBS

To dry, herbs should be bunched in small quantities, and hung on strings in airy places, or put in brown paper bags, the bags of thin paper, or placed in baskets hung in airy places. Herbs can be dried on tables, the tables spread with sheets of paper (not newspaper), or on fine-mesh wire netting, and covered with cotton gauze to protect from dust. Never use plastic, neither as bags nor as sheeting. Plastic excludes air and holds dampness. Do not dry in full sunlight because strong sunlight over-dries herbs and reduces their medicinal properties. In damp and sunless climates gentle heat can be used. A modern, bad development in the herbal trade is quick drying by electricity. This is worse than sundrying. Electricity-dried herbs are over brittle, lack their natural scents, and are very reduced in medicinal properties.

Herbs when fully dried should be stored in strong-textured bags of brown paper, the herbs not packed too tightly into such bags. Or strong cotton bags can be used. If cotton bags are not obtainable, then new cotton pillow-cases, of small, single size, can be used. The necks of paper or cotton bags should be well twisted to exclude all air and to prevent the entry of the smallest insects, and then very firmly tied with string or pieces of elastic. In the storing of herbs precautions need to be taken, not only against insects such as moths, weevils, ants and others, they must also be kept out of reach of rodents, all of which are likely to eat up (or merely spoil with contamination) our stores of medicinal herbs.

In lands where sunlight is very infrequent and the climate is very damp and cold, then a luke-warm oven can be used. This is different from the use of electric machines for drying herbs. Only very mild oven heat is required and the drying done very slowly with the door of the oven kept partly open.

TO MAKE HERBAL BREWS AND PILLS

The *Standard Infusion* used throughout the medicinal treatments now advised is made as follows:

Take one large handful of the fresh herbs (or two tablespoons of the dried herbs) and cut up small if the herbs are of large leaf or flowers.

Place the herbs in a pan which has a tight lid (the lid prevents the loss of aromatic properties of herbs) and pour over the herbs one pint of cold water. Then heat slowly on a low flame and remove from heat before boiling-point is reached. Be watchful when heating, as boiling spoils the medicinal properties of herbs. When sufficiently heated, remove from the heat and stand to brew for several hours. Keep the pan lidded during the brewing. Brew for three or four hours.

Then pour the cooled, brewed herbs into a glass jar.

Cover the top of the jar with a circle of paper or cotton cloth, to exclude dust but not to cut off air.

Herbal brews are living liquids, if tightly capped they will go sour very speedily. Despite proper ventilation, herbal brews will not keep fresh and usable for longer than several days, and a mere one day during hot weather. Watch out for bubbles in the herbal brews, that means there is fermentation and they are no longer fit for medicine. General dose is one dessertspoon of the brew given morning and night.

Pills can be home-made, using fresh or dry herbs. The herbs need to be finely cut, and when in dry form they are best reduced to a powder. Bind the herbs into pills by rolling them in a mixture of honey and flour. Thick honey is easier to bind pills than is thin honey. Make the herbal pills into a paste, then break them up into small pills of a size that a cat can swallow (very small pills are needed for kittens). A pill the size of a large pea would be suitable for adult cats and smaller for kittens.

Dosing of cats and kittens

Cats are much more difficult to dose than are dogs. That is really a good thing for cats, as in that way they save themselves from over-much medication. Of course when medicine is given in that bad form of an injection, using a syringe, then the cat cannot save itself from over-medication. In my half century of veterinary work, I have never once used a syringe on any animal. Totally unnatural! Injections bypass all the protective powers of the animal, present in the mouth and throat, and they bypass all the immune system's danger signals given when medication is in progress.

However medicines are needed sometimes for our cats, especially are they needed to remove worms if the cat should become infected. Presentday, because the earth is so dirty, soured by impure air and polluted rain, worms are alarmingly on the increase in man and animal.

As I have just written, cats are difficult to dose. Therefore they should be trained to accept fluids and pills put into their mouths when they are still young kittens. To train kittens to pills-taking, make fake giving of pills and medicines, using for the former merely tiny pieces of flour and honey, and for the latter merely water and honey. Pat and praise the kitten when it accepts and swallows its medicine!

Pills are merely pushed down the throat, with one finger. Fluids are given in a small plastic spoon or bottle, which does not feel cold or hard in the mouth.

Signs of illness

Medication is often conditional on the pulse beat and the temperature. The pulse is taken by finding that main artery which crosses the inner thigh. Press that artery with one or two fingers, on to the bone, and then count the pulse beats. Pulse beats of the cat are more rapid than the dog, the dog's pulse in normal health being 90–100 beats a minute, while the cat has pulse beats of 110–120 to the minute. The temperature also may need to be taken, and again the temperature of the cat differs from the dog. The cat is usually about 102°F, compared with the dog's normal more constant temperature of 101.4°F. The temperature of dogs is usually taken by inserting the thermometer mercury end into the anus, but the cat, being much more nervous, should have its temperature taken by holding the thermometer in place in the pit of the forearm.

If a thermometer is not available, the presence of fever can be detected quite well by feeling the inner sides of the ears. If merely warm, the cat is all right, if very hot, fever is then indicated, and the cat is ill with one ailment or another.

Another simple way of knowing if a cat is sick, is scrutiny

of the eyes: eye diagnosis. In normal health the white areas of cat eyes are a clean white. In sickness the area becomes reddened. Also, the inner lids of the eyes, which are normally a pale pink, are very red. Further more, the pupils lose their brightness and become dull-looking. In sickness the breath also changes, becomes fetid instead of clean-smelling.

Internal cleansing

As I have already said, I am limiting the cat ailments to the common ones of the feline race. The basis for treatment is much the same for most of the canine ailments and that is simple internal cleansing with the herbs most famed for this purpose, especially garlic, southernwood and sage, and the use of pure honey, which I have pioneered as a life-saving medicine (as well as food) for animals of all kinds.

I am not really differing in what I recommend from some of the greatest of our healers, the ancient ones. First there is Hippocrates, the great Greek doctor, called the Father of all Medicine, and followed to this day by wise healers. Hippocrates cured all the ailments of humans with two basic remedies, Hydromel (honey and water) and Oxymel (vinegar and water). He made such wise edicts as, 'Let food be your medicine, and your medicine be your food.' He also said, 'Give me a high fever in my patient and I will cure any ailment.' Hippocrates understood the valuable, curative purpose of a fever; it is there to burn up the invading bacteria causing the ailments, whereas the modern doctor is mainly concerned with quick reduction of a fever using unnatural medicines, thus prolonging the ailment and possibly killing the patient! Hippocrates also taught that 'Fresh air is the most important nutriment.' Therefore remember that, when treating a sick cat, try and provide fresh air: open the windows, even though the outer air may be typical city polluted, it at least provides some change of air indoors.

The American veterinary surgeon, Dr Richard Pitcairn, whose book I have already mentioned, in his chapter on 'The Holistic Approach and Alternative Therapies in Veterinary Medicine', writes of my herbal work:

> Herbal remedies have been successfully used to treat many illnesses in animals throughout the centuries. In recent years Juliette de Baïracli Levy has popularized their use for this purpose in her detailed writings (which also emphasize the importance of natural diet and fasting). She has reported successful results in the treatment of the following common problems, mange, distemper, kidney and bladder trouble, arthritis, anaemia, diabetes, lepto-spirosis, obesity, wounds and fractures, constipation, diarrhoea, jaundice, heart disorders, warts and cataracts.

I intend in this book to advise on most of those listed ailments, plus a few others which have become prevalent in cats presentday.

EXTERNAL AILMENTS CAUSED BY INSECTS AND PARASITES

I am beginning with the listing of external ailments caused by insect or fungoid parasites, for the presence of these creatures or fungoids can be classified as ailments because of the discomfort they cause. Indeed their presence in very large numbers can cause death: their basic purpose was to kill off the unfit animals which they parasitized. They can kill by the amount of blood that they suck, or cause endless discomfort in irritation and sores. The mange parasites are especially harmful, but fleas and ticks can also prove truly dangerous if they become present in large numbers on any type of animal, not only on cats.

EAR MITES   Mites are classed as *acari* (the word for mite, acarus). They are minute insects of a spider type, and their presence causes much irritation whether within the ears or on other parts of the body. If ear mites are present in large numbers they can so inflame and irritate the ear nerve-endings at the base of the ear canal, that bouts of fits may occur in dogs as well as in the more sensitive cat. There is often internal discharge and a fetid smell.

Ear mites should be taken very seriously, and the infected cat given immediate treatment. Ear mites can be seen by the naked human eye, but with difficulty. A magnifying-glass should be used to make identification more sure, as it is possible to confuse ear mites with common canker of the ear, the latter being a much less serious problem. The irritation caused by ear mites may cause further harm to the cat, because the cat often bangs its head on the floor or against hard objects, trying to alleviate the irritation within its ears.

Treatment   Either use a strong brew of wormwood and rue, equal parts, a teaspoon of each herb to several tablespoons of water. Pour the water cold on to the herbs, then heat, keeping covered with a lid; remove from the heat just before boiling point and stand to brew for several hours. To each teaspoon of this brew, add one or two drops or spirit of oil of eucalyptus. Note, a few drops only, as eucalyptus is very burning and could madden the cat if the dose is over-strong. If even one drop causes much upset to the cat, then immediately put into the ear a small amount of fresh milk. (Fresh milk neutralizes all burning things speedily.) Allow the brew to remain in the ear for five minutes or so, gently massaging the base of the ear with the hand. Both ears must be treated, even if only one ear is infected. (This rule applies to all ear treatments and also to eyes because both are closely linked.)

Now soak pieces of cotton-wool in witch-hazel spirit

(extract) obtainable from all good pharmacies. Wind these cotton swabs around scissors with long blades, and thus gently get the witch-hazel-soaked cotton swabs into the ear. Move the swabs gently to and fro to mop up the discharge and also any ear mites which may have survived the herbal brew. Burn the swabs after use, and use a fresh swab for each ear.

Further treatment: give garlic internally, to improve the condition of the entire cat body because ear mites are more apt to trouble unfit animals.

Mites are also the cause of the very troublesome and highly infectious maladies known as mange, and which are of two kinds, sarcoptic and follicular.

SARCOPTIC MANGE   This skin ailment is very infectious and rapidly spreads from cat to cat, also to other animals such as dogs and rabbits. The mange mites are too small to be seen other than under a microscope. Loss of hair results from their presence, and there is intense irritation of the skin. Sarcoptic mange can also be transmitted to humans.

The severe inflammation, also formation of pustules and unpleasant odour, distinguish sarcoptic mange from common eczema. Microscopic examination of skin scrapings will confirm mange, the mites then being detected.

Internal treatment is as important as external. Indeed, Dr Pitcairn believes that improving internal health can cure the ailment without any other treatment in many cases.

As for all ailments of the parasite class, use protective dieting, making the skin and the bloodstream unattractive to the attempted invasion of parasites. Give internally much garlic, also red (strong) pepper. Both can be given as pills or capsules if the cat objects to their taste in food. These pungent herbs linger in the bloodstream and also penetrate the skin, making both unpleasant-tasting to the would-be parasite invaders. Avoid sugar in the diet because a sugar-rich bloodstream is attractive to all parasites including mosquitoes, lice, fleas and ticks.

Treatment Internal: as advised above, using pungent herbs in the daily diet. Also a short fasting treatment may be helpful, with a nightly laxative. (See Internal Cleansing Treatment, later in this chapter, for a suitable laxative). External: make strong lotions from the following fruit and herbs.

Lemon Fruits Lotion This is one of the most effective treatments for both types of mange. Save all lemon fruit halves and place them in a gallon container, nearly filled with cold water, at least twenty-four halves to one gallon. In hot climates sun-infuse the lemon halves, in cold climates pour hot water over them. Let the lemon halves remain for days in the water until they turn mouldy, then replace with fresh halves. Before removing the old lemon halves squeeze them very strongly into the container, then add the new lemons. To make the lemon lotion stronger, add the juice of at least two lemons to the lemon-peel water. Keep the container covered against dust and insects by using a sheet of strong paper, not waxed paper, or use a cotton cloth.

Rub this lotion into every part of the cat's body daily. A little can be rubbed inside the ears. Continue the treatment until the case is cured.

Garlic Lotion Mince up six whole roots of garlic, at least forty garlic cloves are needed. The garlic can be infused in white beer or in water. One cup of either to every root of garlic. If water is used, then it needs to be at boiling point when pouring it on to the garlic. Keep the lotion covered with strong paper to prevent evaporation of the essential oil of garlic. Use the garlic brew as advised for lemon.

Caution concerning garlic: use the whole garlic cloves for internal use. Do not use the popular modern garlic oil in capsule form. It is unbalanced and is also an internal irritant. Man can never improve on nature, and garlic when used should be in its whole, natural form.

Bitter Herbs Treatment   A brew of bitter herbs deeply penetrates the skin, and the taste and smell make the skin unpleasing to the mange parasites. Take a handful each of the following herbs: wormwood or southernwood, rue, rosemary, sage. Or take two tablespoons of the same herbs in dry, powdered form. Place in a large pan, with lid, pour over herbs one quart of cold water. Heat slowly, keeping pan tightly lidded to prevent escape of the volatile oil of these herbs. Simmer at boiling point for approximately three minutes, then remove from heat and, keeping the lid on, stand to brew for several hours. Bitter herbs can also be infused in white beer. The boiling of the herbs is not forbidden when the brew is for external use, and one does not need to retain its delicate herbal powers for internal use. Externally one wants the herbs as strong as possible in taste and smell to bring discomfort to parasites or bacteria. Do not strain this herbal brew; leave the herbs in the pan and keep the pan lidded. If the mixture ferments it does not matter as it is only for external use. Rub the mixture into the body skin from head to toe. Also apply to the insides of the ears.

Repeat the herbal application daily until a cure is achieved. Internally give garlic pills, or pills made from the herbs used in this brew. One teaspoon of the mixture, made into pills with flour and honey, to be given morning and night.

Before commencing any of these treatments, the mange case needs to be thoroughly bathed, so that the various treatments can be applied to as clean as possible a body.

FOLLICULAR MANGE (also called DEMODECTIC MANGE)   In this form of mange the mites live in the hair follicles – hence its first name, follicular mange. This is one of the most dreaded feline and canine ailments. The case often becomes almost hairless as the mites destroy the hairs in which they live. The skin often thickens and turns a greyish colour and is known as 'elephant skin'. There is also an unpleasant odour, known as 'mousey'. A further development is a rash of pimples, making the case look as if it has been sprayed all over with gunshot. Cases of follicular mange are often destroyed as being incurable, and this applies to dogs as well as cats.

Follicular mange *is* curable, however, and I have had much success with cases condemned to be destroyed.

Treatment Use any of the treatments given for sarcoptic mange (see above). I would give preference to the garlic or the bitter herbs lotions.

Important note: All bedding must be washed and changed frequently, and cat boxes or baskets must likewise be well cleaned with boiling water. If the cat wears a collar it must be cleansed by rubbing very well with a good leather polish.

American veterinary doctor Richard Pitcairn warns that orthodox treatment for mange is 'harsh, poisonous and generally futile'. And my great teacher, Professor Edmond Bordeaux Szekely also warns that orthodox treatments for all types of ailments of man and animals, when unnatural chemicals are used, are often more dangerous in their effects than are the ailments for which they are being used.

As follicular mange is such a greatly feared, bad and painful ailment, and too often classed as incurable by vets and the cat then put down, I shall give now a report on one of my many successes with the disease. This is the only testimonial I shall give in this book, as if I start on testimonials it will no longer be a handy size, but an expensive volume. Those who want testimonials as to the value of herbal veterinary treatments can find many in my other (longer) veterinary herbal books, *The*

Complete Herbal Handbook for the Dog and Cat, and *The Complete Herbal Handbook for Farm and Stable*, both published by Faber and Faber.

Follicular mange cure of a whippet bitch, UK registered, UK Kennel Club, Laguna Lady Lightfoot. Owner, Mrs Leah Gut of Wangen bei Olten, Switzerland. Mrs Gut purchased this bitch in England and follicular mange developed in a severe form. Leading professional veterinary advice was, arsenic treatment would be needed for at least one year, but cure was unlikely, and, furthermore, this bitch was not to be bred from as her offspring would all likely be infected with follicular mange.

Mrs Gut declined arsenic treatment and instead put the whippet on to my bitter herbs in alcohol treatment, given on page 67. The follicular mange was cured within a month and the bitch's condition was so good Mrs Gut was able to show her in several of the UK's big shows, where she won well. One of the UK judges was the famed Bill Siggers, who found Laguna Lady Lightfoot in 'excellent condition of health'. On return to Switzerland the bitch was again shown, won very well, and became a champion. She won in both Switzerland and Italy. There was a demand for pups from her and she whelped several litters, with show champions in all of them, and not one of her pups developed mange of any kind, neither sarcoptic nor follicular.

Mrs Gut used alcohol to infuse the bitter herbs. I do advise this alcohol infusion for dogs. It can also be used for cats, but it is rather strong. I recommend you to try the bitter herbs hot water infusion first for treatment of cats suffering from both forms of mange.

TICKS These skin parasites are of an order known as *Ixodidae*. They can trouble humans as well as animals and birds of all kinds. They are more prevalent on dogs than on cats, but they *do* parasitize cats and are very troublesome as they often leave painful sores where they have been sucking blood. However the tick is not permanent on its host, it is merely there to suck blood after which it drops off to lay its eggs for the hatching of more ticks. These new ticks wait around for prey such as dogs and cats and attach themselves, especially choosing the ears (inside and outside), around the mouth and around the eyes (where they are very painful and difficult to remove). They are also painful and prevalent on the feet, between the toes.

In addition to living in vegetation, waiting for suitable prey to pass by, ticks can also infest human dwellings, and they will be seen climbing up walls where they hide in wall cracks and behind pictures.

Treatment First should be prevention, and that is regular dusting of the cat with bitter herbs in fine powder form, those same herbs advised for treating the mange mites. A swab of cotton wool can also be soaked in bitter herbs citronella brew, with some drops of eucalyptus oil and citronella oil, and the cat's head and body lightly rubbed with that partial prevent-ive. Avoid the eyes and the genitals when eucalyptus is used: it is very burning.

Ticks are very persistent and long surviving. They bury their heads deeply into the skin while they suck blood. Blood-swollen to a large size, they then drop from the body of their host to lay their eggs, and will then return for a further blood-feast.

To remove a tick with its head firmly buried into the flesh of a cat or other creature, dab the tick body with a drop of paraffin, or a drop of eucalyptus. Those burning substances will cause it to loosen its hold! Some people will actually burn a tick to make it withdraw its head, and they do so by lighting a match, blowing out the flame, and at once applying the hot match-head to the tick body. If the ticks are broken off leaving the head embedded in the skin, a painful sore, or even an abscess can result, therefore always take care to remove the head.

Keep the cat bedding very clean so as not to harbour ticks, and if cats are given freedom of garden and field, frequently examine them for ticks on their return home, to prevent the ticks from establishing themselves in the home.

Ticks are not removed by bathing, as their heads are within the skin and therefore they do not drown. Remember this, and disturb them by use of bitter herbs internally and externally. Given as pills, such herbs make the blood seem unattractive to the would-be blood-suckers; external application to the skin gives it a bitter taste.

LICE   There are many types of lice. They are insects possessing ability to suck blood, and to glue themselves to the skin of their host creature. They are wingless and slow of movement, but if not checked they can become present on a host animal in large numbers, causing much loss of blood and much irritation of the skin. (They are not of the same type as head-lice, now so prevalent on humans.)

Treatment   To remove lice, apply the same treatment as given for ticks, also follow the same prevention. Comb daily with a fine-toothed lice comb. As with ticks, lice are not removed by bathing, but a frequently bathed cat, with resultant very clean hair and skin, will be far less attractive to lice than would be a neglected animal with dirty hair and skin. Bathing also helps remove the eggs of lice which, unlike ticks, are laid on the hair of their hosts.

Lice, similar to ticks, will hide themselves away in human dwellings if not prevented from doing so. Prevention of lice in homes is the same as advised against ticks. Home watchfulness and cleanliness and especial care given to the bedding used by cats are very important.

FLEAS Fleas have the classification of *Arthropoda*, which means jointed foot. The legs area of fleas are responsible for their nuisance power and for their ability to survive so well despite all precautions taken against them. The legs of fleas are capable of endless jumping, and that way they escape from people trying to catch them!

Rats and mice spread fleas among cats and dogs. And it should be remembered that a bite from a rat flea can cause bubonic plague.

I have already told that the rat was put in the Ark by the Devil. I always feel that the flea is also a creation of the Devil and came along hidden in the hair of the rat!

The flea is a truly devilish parasite, so cunning in its persistence to survive all attempts to eradicate it. Fleas trouble humans as well as animals of all kinds, and furthermore they spread that dangerous internal parasite the tapeworm!

Fleas are not content with making their host miserable with their ceaseless biting, and the intense irritation that their bites cause to their victims, they also carry the larval form of tapeworm, and when the dog bites at the irritating flea, and swallows it, the tapeworm develops within the dog, and thus the tapeworm peril spreads (tapeworms the most destructive internally to their hosts, of all the many varieties of worms).

Thousands of pounds are spent annually by cat and dog owners in trying to combat the flea, with little success. Fleas persist and are on the increase, helped by modern pollution of the air which makes skin and hair less clean and more suitable for flea infestation. Also there is presentday unnatural warming of the world's climate.

The cat flea is very similar to the rat flea in size and colour. It is known that the rat flea bites humans, so does the cat flea, which is much more troublesome to humans than is the dog flea. The dog flea is big and brown and therefore is easier to detect and kill than are most species of flea.

Treatment   The best remedy against the cat flea is ceaseless cleanliness of the cat. A daily brushing and combing (using as a comb the finely toothed lice comb), and regular dusting with powdered bitter herbs to make the cat hair unattractive to fleas. Such herbs are totally non-toxic if the cat should lick them off when cleansing itself. This licking of hair points to the importance of never using toxic chemical flea-killers on cats. Cats are very allergic to chemical poisons, including chemical bathing products: such have killed off, painfully, thousands of cats.

I have advised Canex bathing block in the past. It has kept my Afghan hounds and other animals free of fleas for over a dozen years. But Canex became increasingly difficult to obtain, therefore I have had to work out a new flea-control method. I give this now, one which has served me very well in care of my many animals, especially my long-haired Afghan hounds.

Make a bathing lotion as follows: take a cupful of any make of washing-up liquid which claims to be 'kind to the hands' (choose the milder kind, such as Palmolive, with a lemon/lime base) and to every cupful of detergent add a teaspoon of oil of eucalyptus; mix very well. If available, use also a teaspoon of citrus oil. Now wet the dog or cat thoroughly, soaking the fur well. Rub half the lotion very carefully into the fur to reach the skin. Do not neglect any part of the body: under the leg pits, the throat creases, under the tail and all parts of ears. *Keep the lotion out of the eyes* (if any should enter the eyes, then soothe at once by pouring milk – fresh milk, not preserved – into them). Now rinse off the foamy application, then apply the rest of the lotion as thoroughly as the first application. Finally, rinse off very well. Partly dry with towels, then stand the bathed animal on a piece of white paper and brush very well to bring the dead fleas out of the fur. Search the animal for any flea which may have escaped the lather; the fleas will be in a feeble state of survival and can be crushed with ease.

This treatment I have evolved works *not* by dangerous poisoning of the fleas, but by foamy suffocation of them! The eucalyptus, pungent and penetrating yet harmless, brings the fleas to the surface of the fur and there they suffocate in the copious foam. That this advised treatment is harmless is shown in the fact (unfortunate!) that ticks and lice, with their heads buried in the skin of their prey, are not killed by this treatment. The fleas do not bury their heads into the skin, they are surface creatures, and thus they are killed.

A note of caution: this treatment has been used, by myself and others, for cats and dogs with great success. But it is for healthy animals, properly raised. Other animals on the common modern feline and canine diet of cooked and conserved food, may have over-tender skin and thus develop irritation following such treatment. I have used it on very young Afghan hound puppies with great success and no skin discomfort.

I am working on a mixture of seven essential herbal and tree oils, repellent to fleas, which will give further protection when applied in the bathing of the cats, further harass the fleas and permeate skin and fur of the cat or dog, thus delaying speedy return of other fleas on to the bathed animal. Such mixture would fortify simple eucalyptus oil. Citrus oil is a proved and useful flea deterrent and killer, especially oil of orange (obtainable from pharmacies). Add one teaspoon of citrus oil to a cupful of harmless shampoo for human babies, and use as a bathing shampoo. Give the cat two latherings before rinsing clean.

Flea collars: these collars to deter fleas are now very popular. They are quite effective, but personally I would never use them on any of my animals as much clinical evidence has shown that they can cause irritation of (and even damage to) eyes. Any product which bears a warning to 'keep out of reach of children' is very suspect to me. The American vet, Dr Pitcairn, totally condemns cat collars in his book, *Natural Health for Dogs and Cats*, 'They don't work. They are toxic.

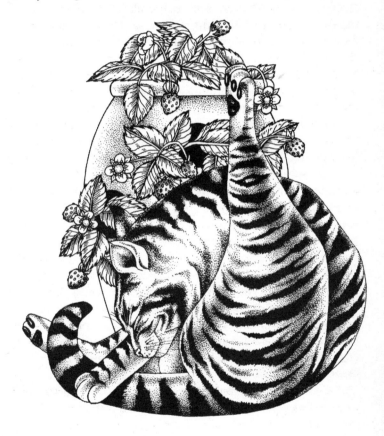

Some cats even hang themselves on them or get the collars caught between their jaws causing serious damage.'

Herbal shops (especially in America) are now supplying anti-flea collars made from herbs, carefully woven, and further impregnated with oils from such herbs, the principal ones being eucalyptus, pennyroyal and rosemary (fleas are said to detest the odour of rosemary). Such collars break easily under pressure, therefore minimize the self-hanging or choking risks for cats. But such collars do not retain their scent powers for long, therefore would need to be replaced with new ones quite frequently. Their merit is that they are harmless to health.

To sum up: remember that the best way to combat fleas is a regular (no failing) daily brisk grooming with brush and use of a fine-toothed comb. This harasses fleas and kills many of them. Further, the use of anti-flea herbs in the form of a fine powder dusted into the coat, also the use of the herbal oils' rub advised against ticks; and finally a regular bathing with a proved *safe* flea-killer product.

Keep the cat bed and its surroundings (floor, carpet) very well cleaned against flea eggs which may be laid there, washing such cat areas frequently with hot water and disinfectant soap, and use of a vacuum cleaner (vacuuming of carpets and furnishings is a sure way of removing flea eggs and thus breaking up the fleas' life-cycle. Fleas lay their eggs away from their hosts and their young hatch out on the ground and are fed by the dried blood which the fleas excrete as 'droppings', those small black grains found on animals infected with fleas. These blood grains fall to the floor and feed flea larvae which when adult jump on to any animal (or person) within reach.

Dried and powdered pennyroyal sprinkled on to carpets where fleas are prevalent, then brushed out after an hour or so, will remove fleas and their eggs. This I was told by a visitor from the USA. The best control I know for fleas' and lice eggs in carpets and upholstery is to dust down with white pepper. May make the cats sneeze but very effective! I use it also against mice and rats in my garden (curry powder and powdered ginger are also useful garden pest deterrents). Another treatment indoors is rubbing carpets and upholstery well with a cloth dipped into a mixture of water and turpentine, the turpentine fairly strong. Never use aerosols.

RINGWORM   This is not a skin insect parasite as are those previously described in this chapter, nor is ringworm a worm! It is a fungus.

There are three species of fungi that parasitize the skin of animals of all kinds, especially cats. These fungi are classified as *dermatophytes*, skin plants, and these plants are spread by contact from ringworm victims, from earth, bedding and clothing, which have had contact with the ringworm fungus.

This fungus, unfortunately, is a very hardy one and can persist for a very long time. Therefore, strong cleansing measures must be taken to overcome ringworm fungus once it has become established in your area. Ringworm is conveyed from animals to humans and vice versa.

Fortunately, by using logic and not especially medicine I have evolved a good cure for this fungus. But first I shall describe ringworm so that it can be recognized if it does infect your cat or cats.

Ringworm is shown as circular patches (rings), which can occur on any part of the body, but especially on the face. This fungal growth starts off at a centre point, then spreads out to make a ring shape. The fungus usually destroys the hair, causing unsightly bald circular patches to appear, usually many inches wide. (On people, the ringworm manifests itself as circular red patches and can appear on any part of the body.)

Treatment Treat as for mange, if widespread. Internal treatment to disinfect the bloodstream (as advised for mange) is also advised. If the ringworm is present merely in a few patches, then the method which I evolved of suffocating the fungus is very effective: to cut off all its contact with air. This is done by painting a glaze over the fungus rings. Pure, fresh-squeezed (not bottled or tinned) lemon juice forms an excellent glaze on the skin, and so does white of egg, applied in many thicknesses to the skin. Another glaze can be provided by nail varnish, but this must not be allowed to stay on the skin over-long, as varnish can crack the skin surface. The varnish should be removed frequently with proper nail varnish remover, and then reapplied before the fungus loses its suffocation treatment. As further part of the treatment, there must be thorough cleansing of cat collar (if one is worn) and cat bedding and surroundings of the cat bed.

EXTERNAL AILMENTS: OTHER SKIN TROUBLES

This ends the section on skin and hair parasites of the cat, but while writing on skin, I shall now continue with other skin troubles, scalds and eczema, both over-frequent for the domestic cat, also abscesses, wounds, splinters, bleeding.

SCALDS Cats are well known to 'get under the feet' of their owners. This is especially likely when owners are carrying good-smelling things from cooker to table. The owner stumbles over the cat and, if hot liquid foods are being carried, the cat very likely will be scalded.

Treatment of scalds must be immediate, no delay. If treated immediately scald scars do not develop. Long-haired cats needs to be clipped in the area of the scald so that the dressing being used can reach the skin.

Treatment   The best-ever for scalds is one I learnt in Spain and it consists of vinegar and honey (the two great remedies of the famed Greek doctor Hippocrates). Bathe the scalded area with pure vinegar, keep applying vinegar for ten minutes, then spread thick honey over the scald areas. Apply the honey in generous amount so as to exclude all air. In all forms of scalds and burns, the exclusion of air is of the utmost importance. Keep applying honey until all pain seems to have ceased even when the scalded area is touched by the human hand. Application of honey, every few hours, may have to continue throughout the day or night.

Another excellent treatment for scalds is given by applying finely-grated raw potato. Wash the potato and then, using a metal grater, grate finely. Then place the potato pulp on the scalded area and hold in place by a cotton bandage moistened in vinegar. Apply freshly-grated potato every few hours.

A third remedy is whites of several eggs applied to the scald or scalds and, as above, bind over with a cotton bandage moistened with vinegar.

Note: burns are treated in exactly the same way, as above. Exclusion of all air is of equal importance. These exact remedies are also excellent for human scalds and burns, because cats 'getting under feet' can also cause scalds to humans when they are carrying hot foods.

ABSCESS   Abscesses can occur on any part of a cat's body, also between the toes, where they are called interdigital cysts. Cats are likely to get more abscesses than are dogs, as they are more likely to get into fights (the males). Their fine claws scratch their opponents, the scratches close up, holding

79

inside them any dirt which may have entered, inflammation and then abscesses result. Thorns and other matter from wild plants also easily enter the fine skin of cats and result in abscesses.

Treatment   Hot fomentation with a brew of blackberry leaves or elder leaves or blossom. Apply the brew as hot as the cat can tolerate, on a piece of flannel. Repeat the treatment three times during the day and once late at night.

An alternative treatment is to macerate several cloves of garlic within the heart of an onion. Heat the onion thoroughly until it has softened, then sprinkle with a little common salt and apply, as hot as the cat will tolerate, on to the abscess, and hold in position with one's hands until the onion has turned cold. Similar to instructions above, repeat the treatment three times and apply one time at night.

A further treatment is raw tomato, in a very ripe condition, pressed into a pulp, skin and all, sprinkled with a little salt and placed on the abscess, then bandaged into place with a piece of cotton cloth soaked in cold water.

WOUNDS   Wounds in cats usually occur from fights, or from being cut by sharp twigs when tree-climbing, or from becoming entangled in barbed-wire fencing.

Treatment   Rosemary herb, leaves and flowers, is the specific treatment for all types of wound. It is a natural disinfectant and a speedy healer. I have treated truly dreadful wounds in all types of animals, merely by frequent bathing with a strong brew of rosemary. One handful of rosemary herb, cut finely, to one pint of cold water. Lid over the pan, heat slowly, allow to boil for a few minutes as it is for external use. With the lid still on, allow to stand and brew for half an hour or so, then bathe the wound with the rosemary. Bathe, as advised above for abscess, during the day and once in the night. If the wound is a deep one and needs to be covered do *not* place a bandage directly on to the wound, first layer the place with cold-water-rinsed green healing leaves of any of the following or with a mixture of several: mallow, geranium (garden not wild), nasturtium, castor-oil leaves (called *Manus Christi*, because Christ used them so often in his healing work in the Holy Land, and the castor-oil shrub leaves do resemble a human hand in their five-finger form), or cabbage (young) leaves. Place a cold-water-dampened bandage to hold the leaves in place and, following each bathing with rosemary brew, change the leaves covering the wound, applying fresh ones.

If a cat injures a leg or foot, give the following treatment immediately: pound up one raw onion of medium size, sprinkle on a little salt. Soak a cotton cloth in vinegar, then spread the onion on to the cloth and wrap around the leg, bandaging firmly so that it will stay in place. This treatment gives immediate pain relief, also cures the sprain or bad bruising. Repeat several times daily and for some days, if the cat still shows pain and continues to limp badly.

SPLINTERS Cats are prone to splinters because they are such active climbers, and will also go into thorny places when hunting prey, and in the home they are constantly using their claws on woody objects. With splinters it is a case of like cures like.

Treatment Make a strong brew of hawthorn or blackthorn twigs, and apply this hot to the place of the splinter. Apply the thorn brew, hot, frequently during the day, or for several days, until the area has softened and the splinter has surfaced. Then remove the splinter, using a thick needle end to prise it out of the flesh, having boiled the needle point to sterilize it first.

BLEEDING With the exception of some dangerous forms of bleeding, which I shall now describe, follow the exact treatments described for wounds.

Treatment Very heavy bleeding from accident wounds: If you are fortunate enough to have available sage plants, pull several handfuls from the sage, crush the herb in your hands and press over the wounds: this is how Spanish hunters treat heavy bleeding, a method which I have used with much success on myself and many types of animals.

Another wonderful wound herb is sphagnum moss, and a supply should be kept in every home for emergency use on people as well as for animals. Sphagnum grows in moorland places where conditions are boggy and when this moss has been dried it can absorb a very large amount of moisture, therefore when applied to badly bleeding wounds it soaks up the blood and helps to check the flow. This moss is also rich in natural iodine and so is antiseptic as well as powerfully absorbent. (Do note that natural iodine is very different from the chemical form of iodine, which dulls the natural healing process and hardens – even burns – the skin and causes formation of excessively coarse scar tissue.)

An ancient method of checking heavy bleeding is to plug the wounds with cobwebs. Cobwebs for use in wounds must be taken from clean places, and any dust must be shaken off them. The spider-webs are then inserted into the wounds. I remember plugging with cobwebs leaking udders of cows in Mexico, their udders having been torn on barbed wire: this use of cobwebs amazed the Mexicans, but was very successful.

Another proved wound herb is yarrow, used as a lotion, following its brewing, likewise comfrey root, which has a unique mucilage content, is excellent to restrain bleeding and is very healing as a lotion.

When there is bleeding from the mouth, the case should be treated for shock, not medicated at all, only placed in a quiet, dim-lit place, and packs of sphagnum, or layers of cotton wool, placed around the mouth to absorb the blood. When signs of recovery are showing, then slowly give, in a plastic bottle, sips of a mixture of lime blossom and vervain (*Verbena*) tea, as a shock remedy, a teaspoon of each to a cup of water, brewed to make a strong tea, sweetened with honey.

When there is bleeding from the ears, fracture of the skull is the likely cause and there is little chance of a cure.

AILMENTS OF THE DIGESTIVE SYSTEM

INDIGESTION When the cat shows discomfort after eating, with hiccups, bloating, coughing, then put on to a semi-fast, giving only watered milk sweetened with a little honey. Small meals of flaked barley (which is internally healing and soothing), soaked in milk or buttermilk can also be given.

Treatment As medicine, give a strong tea made from dill seed and camomile herb, one teaspoon of each to every cup of warm water. Give also charcoal tablets, cut small for getting them down the cat's throat. Make sure the charcoal tablets are made from vegetable charcoal and not from animal bones. The latter is far cheaper, but is of very limited internal purifying power.

DIARRHOEA, DYSENTERY Fast for several days, allowing only weak honey-water, and improve this water by use of the curative herbs, dill and camomile.

Treatment Follow this fasting with healing meals made from barley flakes, slippery elm flour, and a little honey mixed into warm milk. Juices of the following fruits, peaches, bilberries, pomegranates are curative: one dessertspoonful of any of these fruits given three times daily. If not available, give rose-hip tea.

Follow on this internal soothing treatment with light meals of steamed or baked fish, sprinkled with finely-cut green herbs, chickweed, parsley, cress, celery, dill or cleavers. Chickweed and parsley are binding in diarrhoea. Buttermilk can also be given. Also raisins, the seedless ones. They absorb excess fluid from the bowels but do not block them. Never try to suppress diarrhoea with chemicals or with clay-type products which block up the bowels. Diarrhoea is a useful cleansing process, let it run its natural course, only help the case by providing a light semi-fast of things which heal and soothe internally, but do not block or harden the intestinal system. As with indigestion, the purifying vege-table charcoal tablets can also be given.

CONSTIPATION This, of course, is the reverse of diarrhoea, just described. There are two prevalent causes of constipation in cats. First, lack of roughage in their diet. In addition, too many bones given frequently in a week are constipating as well as wearing down the teeth over-much. (Wolves some-times have tooth problems from much eating of bones; their teeth get worn down and they then cannot kill their prey effectively.)

However, the major reason for constipation in house-confined cats is that their owners do not pay sufficient atten-tion to the cat's litter-tray. Cats have a very sensitive power of scent, and they object to bad odours. As cat excreta has an unpleasant smell, animals will delay having to excrete on a dirty litter tray, and so become constipated.

Treatment Increase the roughage in the diet by giving many times in the week a dessertspoon of finely grated raw carrot, a teaspoon of grated coconut, and a teaspoon of raw bran (not commercial-type bran sold in fancy packets). If you can obtain that sesame-concentrated product known as tahina (sold in many health food shops) then add a teaspoon of that to the diet.

Replace daily the litter in the litter trays. Sprinkle this with ash from a wood fire if available, or collect from the country-side a quantity of pine needles and add a handful of pine daily to the litter tray.

In cases of severe constipation, when the cat seems to have great difficulty in excreting at all, then dose with senna pods (using the large variety). Two senna pods to two large tea-spoons of water. Soak all day, then give at night, adding a pinch of powdered ginger to prevent the pods from griping (griping is a problem with senna). A little honey can be added to the senna water, as it tastes unpleasant. Of course only the infusion, not the pods, is given.

Finally, concerning constipation, it should be emphasized that if cats are compelled to use dirty litter-trays, they will probably delay excreting for long periods, thus harming the natural nerve signal to excrete when the bowel is ready to empty itself. This, in time, could result in bowel cancer.

FELINE PANLEUKOPENIA (also called FELINE DISTEMPER, INFECTIOUS ENTERITIS, FELINE TYPHUS). This is the most frequent feline ailment and their greatest killer. In truth it is an advanced, far worse, form of common cat distemper which, purpose-sent by Nature, was to cleanse the felines of toxic internal accumulations. But presentday, with feline health greatly on the decline due to *un*natural diet and the general lack of exercise, this disease has developed into a very severe one indeed. It is less common among country-living cats, but is a veritable plague among the town-dwellers. The disease develops very suddenly, with little pre-warning. When young kittens have lost their short time of disease immunity given to them from their mother's milk, they will have little resistance to this virus, and may die within two days. (Do not despair! Nature-raised kittens are not likely to develop this disease at all.)

It is not known for sure how this disease is transmitted, though it is believed to be taken from the saliva drips, or from vomit, or from urine and excreta of infected cats, deposited on the earth or on grass, or even on street pavings. It is likely also to be carried by houseflies. Anyway, this disease spreads fast and epidemics are frequent.

First symptom of Panleukopenia is a very elevated temperature. The normal cat temperature of around 101.5–102.5°F increases to 105°F, or even higher. The cat becomes very lethargic, the eyes sink into the face, the head hangs as if its neck cannot support it, and the body quickly begins to appear very hydrated.

The ailment worsening, the cat then begins to vomit, first clear watery vomit, then yellow with liver bile or, yet worse, streaked with blood. The cat has a fetid smell.

Treatment There is only one basic treatment and that is of the wild, fasting the cat. Wild creatures have one supreme law; when they are ill or injured they go into hiding in some quiet and dark place, preferably a cave or some deep bushy thicket (preferably of a prickly kind, so that they cannot be attacked by some hunter animal when they are in a weak state and unable to defend themselves). In this chosen solitude the sick creature fasts from all food, may even have to abstain from water, if water is distant and no rain falls. In this fasting time the body and its immune system can concentrate all its powers on overcoming the invading disease bacteria, carrying out a powerful internal self-cleansing. Its body powers are not diverted for the always major task of food digestion (food is not needed at such critical times), and those powers can fully concentrate on curing the ailment. A cat can survive several weeks merely on water. ('Fast and pray' the greatest of the healers, Jesus Christ, taught the sick, and miracles were achieved.)

For medicine: The following are required – a supply of senna pods, powdered ginger, raspberry-leaf tablets, rose-hip tablets (preferably those two herbs combined as one tablet), slippery-elm bark powder, flaked barley.

First, do *not* try and reduce the fever. Remember those words I have already quoted of the great doctor, Hippocrates: 'Give me a high fever and I will cure an ailment.' Sick creatures (animal *and* human) generate a fever to burn up the invading bacteria and when high fever is present the case does not care to eat food and likes to sleep, fasting and sleep being great self-healers.

Immediately prepare a dose of senna pods. (For preparation of senna laxative, see above, under Constipation.) Give the senna nightly, while any fever is present.

Every early morning give two raspberry/rose-hip tablets, two tablets if they are combined, or one of each if they are not combined. These tablets supply a concentration of vitamin C, much needed in this ailment.

Instead of ordinary water, use barley water, made by pouring hot water over flaked barley, a cupful of barley to a pint of water, water kept well below boiling heat. Steep the flakes in the water for several hours and then drain off the water; reheat this barley water to tepid heat only, and then stir in one dessertspoon of honey.

Give no other food until the temperature returns to normal. Then slowly introduce flaked barley, well liquefied in warm milk and sweetened with honey, for several days. Then also lightly steamed on baked white fish (not mackerel) midday and evening meals. Later steamed or roasted chicken can be given.

An important *warning*: after prolonged fasting the cat will be hungry. For the first few days allow only very small portions of solid food, an approximate four tablespoons of solid food per meal. Overeating following a fast can distend the stomach so dangerously that the case can die. (In the concentration camps of the Nazis, thousands of people died from overeating when rescued, their former starvation diet replaced too hurriedly by large meals of heavy foods.)

FELINE (INFECTIOUS) PERITONITIS   This is an ailment of the stomach area and is indicated by vomiting, obvious stomach colic pains and high fever. Kittens do not develop this ailment to the extent of the previous ailment, Panleukopenia, but some do succumb.

Treatment   Exactly as described for Panleukopenia, but omit the senna laxative. For medicine, sprinkle powdered ginger into the barley/honey-water, to calm colic pains, ginger to be a mere pinch only, put into the liquid, as it is very strong. Further, make a brew of mallow leaves and roots, a large handful to a half pint of water. Allow to steep, then squeeze the resultant mucilage into the barley/honey-water and later into the barley/honey/milk fluid. Give vitamin C tablets, as described for Panleukopenia.

In both these serious feline ailments, do remember that an essential part of the treatment is the provision of a well-shaded and quiet place where the cat, fighting for its survival, can rest undisturbed.

WORMS

Having dealt with the ailments of the digestive system, worms are a logical follow-on, as it is in the stomach and digestive tract of cats that worms live.

The remark that I gave concerning the dangers of modern unnatural medicines (often poisonous chemicals), the quote from the wise sayings of Professor Edmond Bordeaux Szekely, that medicines given often, do more harm than the ailment for which they are being used, very surely applies to modern worms treatments. Even such a killer as arsenic is often used in worms medicines. I have never used other than natural remedies in prevention and cure of worms of all kinds (including heartworms in dogs) and have had true success.

First, aim at the prevention of worms. Worms are conveyed to cats from many sources such as: with the milk of their mother (round worms in the form of eggs); the kitten or adult cat that has many fleas, and biting at them swallows them together with the tapeworms of which fleas (despite their smallness) are active carriers in the form of the dried-up tapeworm segments, which then within a host animal will develop into a complete worm; the eating of young rabbits, gophers, and other wild animals; also eating birds such as grouse, which are often infected with tapeworm; the intake of worm eggs direct from infested ground, from places where worm-infected other animals, fellow cats or dogs or wild creatures have left their excreta.

Types of worm infecting the cat: round worms, thread-worms, whip worms, tapeworms. There are other parasitic worms within our domestic animals, but not usual to the cat, therefore I will deal only with the common types of feline worm. In any case, treatments for expelling all types of worm are similar, and any one of them can be followed for any type of worm. Only tapeworm treatment is rather specific, as one has to cause the worm to loosen its head hooks by which it holds on to the stomach or intestinal tract of its hosts; usually it is the intestine.

I can say, from long experience, that if you nature-raise your cat or cats, especially if you are able to do so from kittenhood, you will never have a worm-infested cat. Your kitten or cat may pick up and develop the occasional worm from the sources I have just now listed, but that can soon be expelled by the use of suitable herbs and a laxative. Your cats must have access to couch grass, which is a principal herb in prevention and cure of worms, and cats and dogs seek out this grass and eat it for that purpose as well as for general internal cleansing.

They will either vomit up the grass, expelling with it bile and also mucus in which worms like to bury themselves within their host, and likewise worm eggs will be expelled (unseen) with the vomit; or they excrete the grass as a bunch, again with much internal impurities, including mucus scraped out with the tangle of grass, and excreted. If your cats do not have access to the countryside, then plant this species of grass in pots which they can visit whenever they have the need to eat such a herb.

Couch grass is also called dog grass because dogs eat it so much. The botanical name is *Agrospyrum repens* or *A. canina*. This grass is considered a troublesome weed of gardens because, once established, it is difficult to eradicate. It is distinguished by its long, tough leaf and by its tough, white roots, which are fleshy and jointed; its flower spikes are brownish and of typical grass-family form. In the USA it is known as crab grass. The roots, as well as the leaves, are highly medicinal, but it is the leaves that cats and dogs seek out and eat in quantity. If you are growing couch grass for your cats in pots in town areas, wash the leaves of the grass clumps daily to remove pollution which one does not want one's cat to take in from the grass.

Prevention of worms Give the queen cat well-crushed garlic cloves in her food when she is in-kitten and when she is breastfeeding her litter of kittens. That way the litter will have early immunity from worms. Never neglect giving the finely-cut green herbs in the daily diet; such prevents and expels worms. Give also a sprinkle of fresh bran on the food as roughage expels worms, as do chewed-up pieces of raw bones expelled by the cat.

Treatment to remove round worms, threadworms, whip worms, add several cloves of garlic to all the meals given, for at least ten days. Give every early morning, before food, two pills the size of a large pea made from finely-cut or powdered southernwood and sage, equal parts of both herbs. Make into pills by binding them with flour and honey; push them down the cat or kitten's throat, gently. Every night give two tablets of vegetable charcoal. Such tablets have to be cut small to enter a cat's narrow mouth. Larkhall Natural Health plc sell Herbal Compound tablets (see page 136).

For infestation by any of these species of worm, fast the kitten for one day, the adult cat for two days, giving water only. Confine kitten and cat to make sure they do not get at any food. Morning of the one or two days of the fast, give herbal pills as described above, but make them stronger by adding hot red pepper powder to each pill. Quantity of red pepper, only enough to cover the *tip* of a teaspoon. Half an hour after giving the pills, give a dose of castor oil: two level teaspoons of oil for a kitten, a level tablespoon for an adult cat. Sprinkle the spoon first with a little water before adding the oil, to prevent the oil from sticking to the spoon. If necessary, if the worms still persist, repeat the treatment given above, on the same days every week for a month.

I recently discovered that mustard powder, made into pills as instructed for the herbs, is an effective remover of the three types of worm just described. A heaped teaspoon of pure mustard powder, made into pills with flour and honey and divided into small balls; half of the pills to be given early morning, the other half late night. Follow the mustard treatment for three days.

TAPEWORM This is a nasty worm and can do much internal damage. It is called tapeworm because it is made up of numerous small segments like a tape measure. At the top of the long line of segments is the head, which has a sucker and a circle of hooks which attach themselves to the inner intestinal tract of its host. Each of the segments is a complete worm. The lower segments fall from the cat host, dry up on the ground or house carpets, waiting to be taken up by the mouth of some animal.

The tapeworm is such an internally destructive worm because it gives out toxic fluids which affect its host, even changing the character of its host, altering its food preferences and making its host irritable of character. To cure a cat of tapeworm it is essential that the head is removed from its grip on the intestine, otherwise the worm will continue to make new segments and thus no cure will have been achieved.

A burning, bitter herbal treatment is needed to cause the tapeworm to loosen the grip of its adhesive sucker and hooked head.

Treatment First prepare the cat by feeding a simple diet which excludes all the foods liked by worms, such as fats, sugar, eggs and all white flour products. Give instead a mono-diet of merely flaked oats with skimmed milk or buttermilk. Fortify the oats with worms-removal items such as finely-grated raw carrot and pumpkin seeds, also being fed raw and finely grated.

Next fast the cat for two days, giving only water. The fasting is quite drastic when one realizes that the cat is not actually sick, but it is better than retaining the destructive tapeworm within it. If the cat seems very upset by the fasting, the meals of water can be modified by adding a teaspoon of molasses to every cup of water and further, a sprinkle of raw bran.

Kittens need a fast of only one day when they are younger than eight months. On each morning of the fast give castor oil, a small, level teaspoon for a kitten, and two level teaspoons for an adult cat. Add a little water to the spoon before pouring in the oil, otherwise the oil is apt to adhere to the spoon.

On the morning of the third day, give a large dose of herbal worm-removal tablets, known as herbal compound, and which contain such bitter things as garlic, wormwood (or southernwood), rue, sage, all in powdered form. A kitten would require three tablets, an adult cat six tablets, as a large dose to shock the worm into losing its internal grip on its host. If such tablets are not available in your herbal shop, then make your own as already described in this book, a teaspoon dose of the mixed herbs before addition of the flour and honey.

An alternative treatment is a teaspoon of powdered pumpkin seeds and hot (cayenne) pepper, made into pills at home. If you possess a bottle of tabasco sauce (that very hot table product) then add a few drops of that to the pills mixture. Cover the pills very well with the flour and honey mixture to ensure that the cat is not maddened by the burning taste! As an alternative, empty gelatine capsules, of the smallest size, can be purchased from a pharmacy, and home-filled with the pumpkin and cayenne pepper: the tabasco sauce could not then be added. Half an hour after dosing with the herbal worm-removal pills, give another dose of castor oil, using the same measures as previously. Then feed a meal of a laxative type to bring out the worm. This meal should be approximately a small cupful for an adult cat, less for a kitten. It should be warm and 'sloppy', of fresh (warmed) milk thickened with flaked oats and slippery-elm powder and a level teaspoon of honey. Feed semi-liquid, not very dry.

The cat, upset by the strong herbal tablets and the castor oil, may vomit up the warm, sloppy meal. If so, wait for a quarter of an hour or so and try again with a similar warm meal, for it is in such a meal that the loosened tapeworm will be swept out of the host body when the cat next passes its stool. This excreta should be carefully examined for expelled tapeworm, using a stick, and making sure that the worm body of segments has not merely broken off and left the adhesive head behind within the body. If there is such failure to remove the head, then the treatment should be repeated in one month's time. I say one month because it is important for success that the worming should be carried out just before and during the time of the full moon. *This applies to treatment of all types of worm*, but especially to tapeworms. Worms are much influenced by the moon, and it is around full moon time that eggs or segments are mainly expelled from the host body. Indeed, if one wants to examine a cat for worms, full moon is the time to watch out to see if species of whole worms, or segments in the case of tapeworm, are being passed.

Finally, do remember that worms like to live and breed in an unclean, mucous-filled stomach and intestines, so keep your cat internally clean and there will not be much danger of invasion by worms. Also keep your cat free from fleas, as they are the foremost carriers of tapeworm to animals and birds.

Do not endanger the life of your cat ever by using harsh chemical (poisonous) de-worming products, such as do more harm to the cat than do the worms themselves.

94

OTHER COMMON AILMENTS

FELINE LEUKAEMIA (FELINE CANCER) It is acknowledged that this severe ailment has, in modern times, reached epidemic rating in domestic cats, whereas it is as yet unknown among the wild felines, though is found in caged felines of the world's zoos. It is far less frequent among country-dwelling cats than those of the towns.

Leukaemia is of rapid development in the cat, once it has established itself. However, the encouraging advice is that it *is* a curable form of cancer, provided that the immune system of the leukaemia case has not been destroyed totally by unhealthy environment and by an unnatural diet of modern, processed cat foods. Prevention of this ailment should be the aim of all cat-owners, by raising the cat as close to Nature as possible, with regard to a whole-foods, raw diet, and provision of a good, natural water supply, fresh air and natural light for most of the day. Also keep the cat distant from colour television sets and microwave ovens, all of which are proved to exude radio-activity as X-rays. In addition, do not allow X-rays to be used on your cat for diagnosing of ailments because X-ray diagnosis *is* dangerous. I have witnessed the sterility effect on a male Afghan hound which had been given X-rays on account of a broken leg.

Symptoms of leukaemia are a fading, anaemic look, colourless gums, general emaciation of the body, general lassitude. When the cancer is advanced, with coldness of the entire body and lack of normal appetite, even usually favourite foods are left uneaten.

Treatment Give immediate dietary aid. Add pure honey to all cereal and milk meals, also add molasses (which is very rich in iron and other minerals), one teaspoon of each per cereals meal. Give cereals only in flaked form, soaked in milk, not to be cooked. Give a clove of raw garlic morning and night. Most cats enjoy the taste of garlic but, if refused, then crush the peeled garlic clove, and press down the cat's throat. Give juice of dark grapes, either from packets or cans, but be sure it is labelled as free from preservatives. Grape juice is now found in most health food stores. If you have your own grapes, then, of course, feed the juice fresh-pressed to the cat. Ration of grape juice: one dessertspoon morning and night. If grape juice is not available, then use instead a sweet, dark grape wine. The specific treatment herbs are cleavers, also called goose-grass, and watercress, both herbs cut very small and added to the food. Lightly steamed nettle is also excellent, and raw turnip finely grated. Give one dessertspoon of all of those when possible.

Leukaemia is a chilling disease so when it is advanced keep the cat warm; place a woollen blanket in its bed and provide a rubber hot water bottle well protected from the claws of the cat by many wrappings of cloth (none of them nylon). Protect against bright light, which is very upsetting when a cat is deeply ill.

Have faith in raw garlic treatment. Remember it is one of the few herbs classed as being 'magic' by those great herbalists, the gypsies, who call garlic *moly*.

VIRAL RHINOTRACHEITIS (FVR) Feline Viral Rhinotracheitis is a rapid, contagious virus ailment of cats and is a painful one. It affects the eyes and the upper parts of the respiratory system.

The eyes become glued-up with a thick discharge and beneath the sealed lids ulcers form on the cornea and often will bleed. Likewise the nose becomes congested with a thick mucous discharge, making breathing difficult. In such pain from eyes and nose the cat appears to want to die to end its ordeal. All food is refused: that is sensible on the part of the cat, and no food should be forced on it.

Treatment Give only drinks of camomile tea, fortified with honey and a little brandy. One teaspoon of honey, one of brandy, to every two tablespoons of camomile tea. Obtain the whole herb, not camomile in teabags. Spoonfeed, or plastic-bottle drip, the camomile brew into the cat's mouth, several tablespoons every four hours or so. Use the sweetened camomile also, without the brandy, for bathing the eyes. Soothe the congested nose, and remove the mucus, also with the camomile, then apply oil of sweet almonds to the nostrils and around the mouth. Give crushed garlic cloves (as advised for cancer) for curative medicine. Finely apply the advice given for cancer (see above as to care of the sick cat), giving warmth and shielding from bright light. Also, as with leukaemia, give grape juice as a general strengthener. Then, when the respiratory congestion has lessened and the temperature is near normal, feed the nature foods already described in this chapter.

BLADDER AILMENTS (Stones and gravel, also irritability and inflammation, also blockage) Cats have a delicate urinary system and are more prone than dogs to the above-listed ailments, especially inflammation of urinary organs, stones and blockage.

Symptoms of bladder and kidney disorders are: abnormal thirst, over-profuse or scanty urination, urine of dark colour, often fetid, stiff gait of the back legs.

Treatment Herbs beneficial for ailments of the urinary system are very many. I have selected those which are among the best and also are easily obtainable. Couch-grass, parsley, cleavers (goose-grass), the 'silk' which is within corn cobs.

Couch grass roots are one of the best herbs for all ailments of the urinary system and are advised for treatment of stones.

97

The roots need preparation different from the usual standard brew of gentle heating. The roots need to be placed in a lidded pan, then well bruised. Use half a pint of boiling water to every handful of the roots. Simmer slowly, keeping covered, and reduce the liquid by almost half from the simmering, then remove from heat and brew for several hours. Strain, sweeten with honey and give two teaspoons of the brew morning and night.

A brew of the silk from within corn (maize) cobs, is prepared by the standard method (slow heating and then brewing), a tablespoon of the mixture twice daily, alternating with the couch grass treatment is famed for its soothing and healing effect on the bladder and kidneys. Amount of cornsilk: two teaspoons to one small cup of water. The water from gently-simmered whole barley grains, strained and sweetened with honey, is rightly an important aid to cure of kidney and bladder ailments. Finely-chopped raw parsley is also a remedy for such problems. Give a teaspoon of parsley once daily. Frequent use of parsley also helps prevent these ailments. Feed the parsley fresh, raw, cut very small, a heaped teaspoon is the daily food.

It should be warned that modern chlorinated water is very harmful to the urinary system. If you have only tap water available, then pass it through a water filter. To treat inflammation or blockage of the bladder, use a softening poultice treatment by placing raw bran on a piece of flannel cloth in a pan, then pouring boiling water over the bran; fold the bran within the cloth, squeeze out excess moisture, and apply to the bladder area at a temperature that the cat can tolerate. Repeat the treatment thrice daily. In chronic cases where there is total blockage of the urethra and bladder, seek immediate veterinary help to apply a catheter to prevent likely death.

POISON The painful death from poisons of various kinds threatens the lives of our domestic animals; the poison danger has greatly increased nowadays. If the pet is house-confined there is then little poison danger, unless such lethal things as moth-balls, poisons against mice, cockroaches and other vermin, are left carelessly around.

An old-type but also excellent, poison remedy, is egg whites. It is known that egg whites take the sting out of scalds and burns; they likewise cool the chemical fire of poison. For cats, whites of three eggs, well whipped, then poured into the mouth. Repeat after a short while. *In all types of poison always seek veterinary aid speedily.* Tranquillizers and anaesthetics are valuable help.

I now list below the commonest poisons which our domestic animals, when outdoors, are likely to meet, and I give their usual neutralizing agents, though if the poison is of a very strong variety, neutralizing will not be very effective. It is advisable to keep in stock all of these neutralizing agents in case of need. They are not expensive, so be prepared!

Strychnine Fed deliberately to animals by cruel humans, or picked up from vermin exterminators which are not protected from the reach of dogs and cats. Remedy: permanganate of potash in solution. A saltspoon of the remedy is given in a large cupful of tepid water. Give slowly via the mouth.

Phosphorus Used commonly in rat and mice poisons. Remedy: a dessertspoon of Milk of Magnesia, given in four tablespoons of soda-water.

White lead From pets eating painted surfaces, especially painted wood. Remedy: Epsom salts in solution. One level teaspoon to one cupful of tepid water.

General treatment For all types of poisons, following the giving of the different antidotes/remedies described above:

there must be immediate removal of all possible of the poison taken in. This is achieved by the use of an emetic to induce rapid vomiting.

A quick emetic is a piece of washing soda (used for clothes-washing). I have always kept some of such soda in reserve. But presentday such soda is replaced by modern soap powders or chemical washing liquids and the soda may not be easy to obtain. One must be sure that the soda available is the genuine thing used for clothes-washing and not some dangerous chemical imitation which would be as dangerous as the poison for which it is being used as a remedy. Beware caustic poison.

A piece of soda the size of a shelled hazelnut, broken into two pieces and then pushed well down the cat's throat is the amount needed for an average-size cat or dog and this should promote immediate vomiting. If unable to obtain soda, another effective emetic is a strong solution of powdered mustard in warm water. Stir a heaped teaspoon of mustard into two dessertspoons of warm water. A further vomit inducer is a strong dose of table salt. Two teaspoons of salt mixed into two tablespoons of warm water.

Then the poison must be further swept out of the body through the bowels. Castor oil is the most rapid of all the laxatives. A dose of two teaspoons of the oil for the adult cat. Give the oil neat, do not mix with any other substance. Remember to add a few drops of water to the spoon before pouring the oil into it as castor oil will otherwise stick to the spoon and not fall easily into the mouth. Continue the all-important internal cleansing laxative treatment by further giving a dose of senna pods every morning for three days following the intake of the poison. (For use of senna pods see Constipation, but approximate senna dose for an adult cat is four large pods soaked in four large teaspoons of water.) The specific poison antidote is discontinued after the first day, but should be given at frequent intervals throughout that first day.

Important: the poison case should be fasted. This emergency is not the time to burden the body with digestion of food of any sort; but a heaped teaspoon of honey can be given three times daily to strengthen the heart and to heal internally the damaged organs of digestion. Thick honey is preferable to the thin form. If necessary, the honey can be made into balls by mixing lightly with a little flour and then pushed down the cat's throat.

Herbal Help: this is obtained from rue or hyssop which should be cut finely and made into pills by binding with flour and honey. One full teaspoon of rue a day, divided into pills of suitable size for the patient to swallow. Giver the rue pills morning and night.

Note: rue is a very strong herb, and should only be given in quantity in emergency such as this. Hyssop is used in a similar way, but a larger amount of the herb is given: a tablespoon daily.

Phosphoros All fats must be excluded from the diet when feeding of the patient is resumed after three days or so. The mixture of fat with phosphorus is dangerous: phosphorus lingers a long time in the system. It also induces a craving for water, which likewise is not a good mixture with phosphorus because it actually 'ignites' the phosphorus internally. But to deprive a frantic animal of all liquid intake would be both cruel and unwise. Therefore make any liquid given a controlled and healing drink by feeding only very thick barley water instead of plain water, the barley water sweetened and fortified with the healing substance, pure honey. Some milk, skimmed of all cream, can be added. To every cupful of barley water, add one level teaspoon of honey and two tablespoons of skimmed milk. Keep the case on this liquid diet for five days or so until signs of recovery are shown. Then follow the special diet given for Feline Panleukopenia.

Arsenic and Cyanide They require different treatments because of the terrible effect upon the nervous system, similar to strychnine poisoning: the jerking nervous spasms are commonly more than the heart can take, and speedy death results. For cyanide the internal system must be washed out, from the mouth downwards, veterinary surgeon help being needed.

Veterinary help should also be sought immediately for arsenic poisoning. Thus the case having been given a rapid emetic and laxative to remove as much of the poison as possible, the case should then be rushed to a vet, to be put under sedation. The case should be given immediate sleep to last while the worst of the poison-induced spasms jerk and contort the body, due to the effect upon the nervous system. When the spasms have become far weaker and the danger of heart failure thus overcome, then specific poison neutralizers can be given and the internal cleansing and soothing treatment can begin.

Vegetable charcoal is very helpful because of its great power as an internal purifier and its ability to absorb impurities of all kinds, including poison. It is the charcoal which is used in water purifiers. Doses of charcoal can be given for all types of poison. Morning and night give two charcoal tablets as sold for human use, making sure that the tablets are vegetable charcoal and not made from animal bone. Break the tablets into small pieces before pushing down the cat's throat.

A recovery warning: remember that all cases of poison need provision of quiet and need to be shaded from bright light. Furthermore, do not let any poisoned animals see or feel the grief of their human owners. The suffering of a poisoned animal does provoke *deep* grief in those who have to witness such cruel pain. It is said in the Bible that not a sparrow can die without all heaven being shaken. What then must be felt when an innocent animal is killed by poison? By voice and caress give the suffering animal courage, do not make it further frightened by subjecting it to human grief.

Remember that poisons are made to kill, that they are deadly, and the more deadly they are the more financial profit they will bring to those cruel persons who make them! Therefore chances of survival for poison victims are slender, but yet are possible.

I have cured many cases of poison of all kinds, many of them my own Afghan hounds. Doubtless helped by their strong health, all my hounds survived after they had eaten rat poison and agricultural poisons. In one case a bitch had fallen foul of an agricultural poison differing from the usual poisons, and although this hound lived only two weeks, she was able to whelp her litter of seven pups and feed them for two days. The litter was saved by hand-raising them: I was determined that their beloved mother should at least live on in her children. With the exception of one pup, the litter showed no sign of poison.

In several of my poison cases when rodent poison had been eaten in the countryside, there was lasting damage to the liver, typical of phosphorus, but although the cases lived for many years there was slow decline in health and they were never again normal. Owners should, therefore, prepare themselves for the possibility of lasting damage if rodent poisons have been taken by their pets, and be prepared to give liver ailments treatment for a long time.

On the more positive side I can report that many cases of poisons of all kinds have recovered fully on the treatments I have advised in this chapter.

LIVER AILMENTS   Unlike the dog, the cat is not very prone
to liver ailments, probably because it does not much like the
fat of meat or other fats and is a more sparing eater than the
dog.

The specific herbs for the liver are the 'bitters', southernwood, wormwood, gentian root, centaury, also blue pim-
pernel which is not a bitter but is the best remedy for
hepatitis.

When a cat is 'liverish' there is discolour of the eye whites;
they turn yellowish, breath is strong-smelling, the coat
'stares', and the excreta is often a near-white colour instead of
the normal brown.

Treatment   The bitters are too strong-tasting to give as a
brew. Make pills from the powdered herbs as listed above, or
from root of gentian. One small teaspoon of any one of the
herbs can be made into pills with honey and flour. Give two
pills three times daily.

BROKEN LIMBS   The bones of cats' limbs are fragile and
breaks often occur. Have a vet set the limb and try and
persuade the vet to use the old-fashioned wooden splints
with cotton bandage. If this is done then one can pour a
strong brew of comfrey roots and/or leaves cold over this type
of setting, which hardens it, and also promotes internal
healing of the break. Give also comfrey tablets, two morning
and night. Two folk-names for comfrey are 'boneset' and
'knitbone': this herb has the remarkable power to do both.
Avoid X-rays, which are dangerous. Decline all use of metal
inserted in the limb to hold the broken bone; this modern
practice is unnatural, and often causes problems. Honey also
helps to make new bone tissue.

EXPERIMENTS ON ANIMALS

Modern man defends his use of laboratory animals with the banal statement that 'human beings are more important than animals'. On whose decision, may I ask? Mankind's, I presume. Note that in Noah's ark very careful provisions were made by God for the survival and care of his animals. Note further, that when God offered to reward King Solomon for his wise and dutiful behaviour as the ruler of the Israelites, Solomon did not choose the likely one of increased power or great riches, he asked instead to be given the ability to understand the speech of the beasts and birds and to be able to speak with them. This was granted to Solomon.

How dare modern man take animals of all kinds, from gorillas and the big cats to small birds and rats and mice, and subject them to all sorts of terrible (usually painful) experiments! Often such tests are out of mere curiosity; one such experiment measures how much burning an animal can endure before it dies from the experience.

Cats are popular experiment victims because they can be confined easily in small space and, because their brains are very sensitive, they show quick reactions to the manifold torture inflicted on them. One of the worst of these I have ever seen was in a photograph and featured a cat. From the cat's head and ears came half a dozen tubes of various lengths. The cat's mouth was clamped open to prevent it screaming and biting. I will never forget the agony in that cat's eyes. Never!

In any case various medicines are very poorly tested, for the very reason that laboratory animals are always under stress because of curtailed (in fact almost nil) exercise, unnatural diet, the threatening and awesome atmosphere in such places, and often the presence of parasites such as ticks, lice, and fleas, which flourish under such conditions, and, above all, stress from lack of companionship.

Another futility is that many human animal experimenters cheat in order to obtain satisfactory (and financially beneficial) results. Cat owners! When parting with kittens make sure they do not get into the hands of the laboratory people, from whose premises there is only death, no return ticket into a free and natural life.

5

Names for Cats

Names according to colour, Black Cats, Black-and-white cats, White or silver cats, Creamy cats, Blue or grey cats, Red, golden, ginger or tabby cats, Speckled cats, Cats with white feet and/or leg markings, Mixed-colour cats, Cats of any colour, Names for female cats, Names for male cats, Calling cats, Suitability of names

Cat names! For years on my world travels I have been collecting them. As I have travelled far and wide since my student days my lists of animal names have come to number around a thousand, with hundreds for cats, which I have found the most intriguing of all the animal names.

Names of cats are more varied than those generally used for dogs, horses, donkeys, goats and other animals. An animal-lover friend of mine in Spain suggested that a book could be written entirely about the names of animals internationally. I shall keep that idea in mind.

When I was coming towards the end of this book I never foresaw that the BBC World Service would just then be presenting a programme on cats by that great poet and philosopher, T. S. Eliot, which included a long passage on the naming of cats. I had thought formerly that this deep interest in the names of cats and other animals was peculiar to myself! At the time of the broadcast, with the usual sea-gale blowing outside, reception was poor, but in that reading of the Eliot

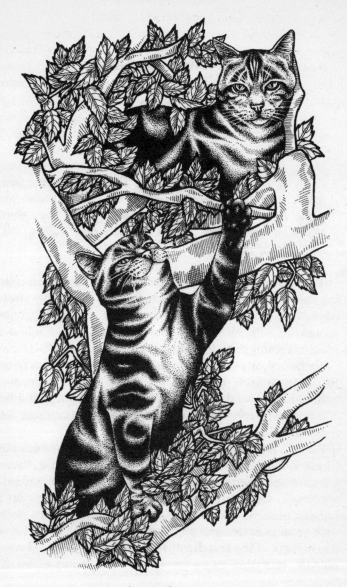

names I don't think I heard one on my list.

In T. S. Eliot's *Old Possum's Book of Practical Cats*, there are several pages of witty and charming poetry devoted to the naming of cats. The publishers, Faber and Faber, have kindly given me permission to make some quotations from *Old Possum* in this book of mine.

Many of the names in my lists in this chapter are unusual, amazing and almost impossible, but none more so than T. S. Eliot's alluring names. In *Old Possum*, he writes:

The Naming of Cats is a difficult matter,
    It isn't just one of your holiday games;
You may think at first I'm as mad as a hatter
When I tell you, a cat must have THREE DIFFERENT NAMES
First of all there's the name that the family use daily . . .
    All of them sensible everyday names.
But I tell you, a cat needs a name that's particular,
    A name that's peculiar and more dignified,
Else how can he keep up his tail perpendicular,
    Or spread out his whiskers, or cherish his pride?

I am enlarging on only a few names on my long list, the first of which is a cat I never met, Felix, whose name is from the Latin, 'happy'. I should, indeed, have liked to have met that far-travelled, valiant cat, for lost in the hold of a Jumbo jet, he travelled the world many times . . . no food, no water. Tail up when found!

I do remember well Madame, a gorgeous, huge, blue, long-haired cat, reclining on a velvet cushion in Istanbul, Turkey: fat, perfumed, adored and, simply, very happy!

Then, Marathon, a giant cat on the island of Icaria, Greece, the biggest cat I have ever seen, like a young tiger for size and strength, but still a domestic cat. The word marathon, we know, symbolizes endurance, from the Greek, and is the name for the crowding anise plants of that land, so difficult to eradicate because of their strong roots.

I have also been told of a cat called Nefertiti and she was never called by anything but her full name. One would have thought a cat with such a regal name to have been sleek and short-haired and of black, or black-and-white colour, stalking about with long-stretched neck, like the bust of the Egyptian queen in Berlin. But this feline Nefertiti was, in fact, small and fluffy and a marmalade colour, but her manner was most queenly and she was obviously very proud of her name.

In the following lists of names I give only the English ones, although many of the cat names in other languages are more musical.

I have not given the very ordinary cat names, and many of which I have known and have given can be classed as nonsensical. But I myself like the unusual in animal names and most of mine are, and have been, so named. Only recently have I heard of a country cat-owner with twenty-eight cats, each one individually named, who at twilight each day would go to the end of her field and call in each one of her cats to be fed.

The most popular names for cats are Tom (Tomi, Tommy) after the male cat, the tom-cat, and Queen (Queenie) after the female queen-cat. I have not included the very common cat names known to everyone, nor to ugly and insulting names such as Devil, Vampire, Satan, Bengi (gypsy for devil), nor the unkind names such as Dunce, Idiot, Simple, Silly, Ugly, all of which I have heard used. Common human names, which are more usual as dog names, Jack, Bill, Bob, Joan, Kate, Betty, and such are not listed.

It is interesting to know that cat names travel. In the book *The Search for Omm Sety*, by Jonathan Cott (Rider), about the two lives of Dorothy Eady (who incidentally confessed that she preferred cats to humans), it is written that 'the common

Irish name for a cat, Maukey, likely comes from the Egyptian word, *mau-key*, meaning "another cat".'

Few foreign names are included in my list, though such names are often more musical than English ones, for instance two names I have given to my hounds in the past, Arcooda (the Greek word for 'bear') and Fuego (the Spanish word for 'fire').

The cat names are not given in alphabetical order as I consider it preferable to classify them loosely according to cat colour, and I have added (M) or (F) when names apply specifically to one sex.

NAMES ACCORDING TO COLOUR

Black cats

Raven, Sooty, Smoky, Dusk, Ebony, Charcoal, Mascara, Shadow, Sweep, Blackberry, Olive, Nepenthe, Shady, Damson, Witch (F), Nocturne.

Black-and-white cats

Magpie, Domino, Motley, Boots (white feet), Piper (Pied Piper), Ludo, Chess, Pierrot, Backgammon (Gammon), Chaplin, Clown.

White or silver cats

Snowy, Snowball, Moony, Daisy, Margarita, Narcissi, Lil, Lily, Lace, Swan, Ghostie, Starry, Sequin, Tinsel, Blanco, Frost, Sugar, Peppermint, Silvie, Diamante, Glitter, Shiner, Gossamer, Cobweb, Gleamy, Stardust, Rain, Rainy, Sleety, Willow, Pusswillow, Snowdrop, Frosty, Blossom, Clover,

Myrtle, Arum, Pearl, Pearly, Lacy, Swanee, Seagull, Egret, Paloma (white dove), Lunar, Turnip.

Creamy cats

Magnolia, Camellia, Curd, Meringue, Yoghurt, Candle, Blondie.

Blue or grey cats

Sky, Turquoise, Lagoon, Lilac, Lupin, Hyacinth, Halcyon, Rainy, Bluey, Gentian, Sapphire, Viola, Iris, Opal, Lazuli, Lavender, Bluette, Bluebell, Kingfisher, Lagoon, Periwinkle, Lapis, Borage, Clary, Dusk, Twilight, Tweedy, Heron, Woodsy, Pigeon, Hazy, Misty, Horizon, Mystery, Sage, Lovage, Teazle, Cygnet, Dove, Azure.

Red, golden, ginger or tabby cats

Flame, Poppy, Ruby, Fiery, Sparky, Peony, Tansy, Mimosa, Jonquil, Goldie, Topaz, Tiger, Ginger, Jasper, Bronzy, Sovereign, Nugget, Farthing, Mango, Harvest, Chanticleer, Handsome, Bizarre, Rouge, Honey, Peach, Coppers, Tansy, Amber, Saffron, Gorsey, Mimosa, Daffy (Daffodil), Marigold, Laburnum, Crumpet, Cookie, Toffee, Candy, Tigerlily, Tigress, Gypsy, Romany, Owli, Owlet.

Speckled cats

Starling, Freckles, Toady, Fritillary, Linnet, Ferrous (his coat was the colour of iron filings).

Cats with white feet and/or leg markings

Socks, Spats, Boots, Garters, Gaiters, Mittens.

Mixed-colour cats

Esmeralda (Esme), Jezebel, Cleopatra (Cleo), Jingle, Jangle, Dazzle, Dicey, Kestrel, Whiskers, Sprite, Spirit, Merry, Mirth, Lynx, Beauty, Lucky, Luv, Herby, Princess, Paisley.

Cats of any colour

Taffeta, Georgette, Treasure, Wonder, Madcap, Shamrock, Marvel, Fairing, Lullaby, Returner, Gadabout, Forester, Enchanter, Wilful, Trick, Can-can (F), Daphne (F), Dainty (F), Cuddles (F), Mystic, Rupert, Tin-can, Busker, Anemone, Always, Clap-clap, Whirler, Perfect, Juniper, Karate, Comrade, Credo, Merman, Beau, Vanity, Bravo, So-so, Rascal, Twinkle, Rosette, Ko-ko, Dandy, Spirit, Buttons, Jewel, Galaxy, Marvel, Lawless, Velvet, Gala, Magnet, Mirth, Roamer, Purry, Brainy.

NAMES FOR FEMALE CATS

Princess, Fantasy, Linden, Sweetie, Secret, Nanette, Stellar, Jemima, Gem, Dreamy, Moth, Rosetta, Velvet, Tiptoes, Go-go, Ballet, Joy, Joybell, Fancy, Flower, Blossom, Posy, Garland, Tiara, Crown, Model, Mamselle, Marilyn, Tambourine, Castanets, Harpy, Lovely, Star, Moonbeam, Milady, Caprice, Carmen.

NAMES FOR MALE CATS

Baron, Duke, Marquis, Prince, King, Kingy, Sultan, Tramp, Rascal, Porgy, Busker, Knave, Ace, Rocket, Pirate, Pedlar, Imp, Comet, Laurel, Joker, Jester, Clowny, Panto, Pan, Goblin, Whiskers, Cupid, Eros, Snazzy, Dandy, Bobbin, Minstrel, Mirth, Beaujangles, Wizard, Guru, Merman, Beau, Bravo, Legend, Legion, Mighty, Monster, Tempest, Hobo, Imago, Brainy, and last of all my son's cat, Frog, such a special and naughty cat, a white with a black moustache.

Calling cats

I also love the name Cuckoo! Although this has a sinister meaning, it makes such a good calling sound, 'Cuckoo! Cuckoo!' and so I have often used this name.

It is important for a cat-owner, when choosing a name for a new cat, to consider how the name *sounds* when called out in gardens or down streets, summoning home loitering cats, also how it blends into apartments.

Flirt, for example, is a sweet cat name, but not a call that one can shout around: it could be mistaken for dirt! Wisteria is pretty name for a silver/blue cat, but when called out could be mistaken for hysteria; Minx could be mistaken for minks, and who wants to be associated with cage-raised animals such as minks, which Nature intended to live wild and free.

Suitability of names

This is something which must be considered carefully to make sure the name fits the cat. It is important not to give a male name to a female cat or the other way round, and not to give a bold name to a timid cat, and further to keep the various colours in cat names for the appropriate cat.

There is much to consider if one is to succeed in choosing a truly suitable name and, most importantly, one which seems to please the cat! Few, for instance, of the names in the various lists would be suitable for dogs.

I do so agree with T. S. Eliot, whom I quoted earlier in this chapter, when he writes, 'The Naming of Cats is a difficult matter, It isn't just one of your holiday games'. He also wrote, 'Again I must remind you that A Dog's a Dog – A CAT'S A CAT.' And,

> When you notice a cat in profound meditation,
>   The reason, I tell you, is always the same;
> His mind is engaged in rapt contemplation
>   Of the thought, of the thought of his name:
>   . . . Deep and inscrutable singular name.

A cat-loving friend looking over this cats' book when in manuscript, declared she would purchase a copy as soon as published, if only to get the cat names! So I hope that, with T. S. Eliot's humour to encourage you and the long list of names that I have collected, despite in many cases their strangeness, you will make a true success of naming that new kitten or rescued 'stray' cat. Happy naming!

6

Conclusion

Return to Nature, Plea for love, Care for cats, Burial of pets, Protection of cats, Treatment of animals, Herbal care, Love your animals, Last words, 'Cats' Eyes'

Now I have reached the end of this book, which always is a good time for the author, and my Afghan hounds always join me in an 'end of book' celebration. Since I have written eighteen books, my hounds have enjoyed much celebrating! (The home-made wine from my grapes, and honey-cake.) Often, when writing this natural health cats' book, I have looked away from my typewriter to my Afghan hounds, and their impressive good health has told me well that this book would be giving good advice to cat-owners, well-proved advice, on how to keep all cats happy and healthy.

My French publishers, Terre Vivante of Paris, wrote on the jacket of my book *The Complete Herbal Handbook for the Dog and Cat* (French title: *Chiens et Chats, leur Médecine naturelle*) that my work is rich in fifty years of experience and that I am the uncontested pioneer of the natural raising of dogs and cats, with books translated into many languages. Their praise is kind and I hope that this new book will help to justify what Terre Vivante wrote about my veterinary work.

Fifty years! Looking back to my student days when I first turned away from chemical- and vaccine-dominated veterinary medicine and turned to herbs, my writings were

ridiculed in the canine journals in which they were published. But Arthur Marples, the editor of England's great
canine weekly journal, *Our Dogs*, praised my work and gave
me space in his journal to write about the healing wonders of
herbs. I was then specializing in canine distemper disease.

Return to Nature

Presentday, one finds a remarkable change in medicine for
man and animals: a return to the natural medicine of herbs, to
the traditional healing plants of the fields and woodlands
instead of from the chemical drugs' laboratories where
experimental animals cower in their cages, sick and fearful
because of the unnatural treatments and medicines which
they are being forced to take – innocent prisoners indeed.

In almost every town of the world today there are
university-qualified vets using herbs or homeopathy to cure
animals of their ailments. Such medicine is called simply,
Alternative Medicine, and the natural immune system
present in every living thing is now given much care and
support, whereas formerly its very existence was ignored.

One may well ask why there has been this return to herbs
and homeopathy. Simply because chemotherapy badly failed
both man and the domestic animals.

Modern books of veterinary medicine are now tomes vast
in size needed to list all the teeming modern ailments of the
animal world, brought about by unnatural medicine and diet.
The wild animals mostly still retain their good health and
their keen intelligence and survival urge, bless them!

Plea for love

I want to plead for more love to be shown to animals, domestic and wild, for never before has their lot been so painful at

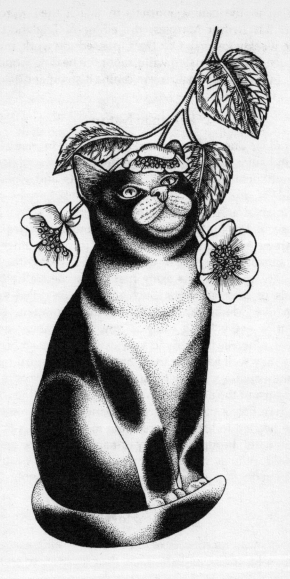

the hands of most of mankind. We find widespread poisoning, trapping and shooting of animals, and there is the terrible plight of the farm beasts, subjected to factory farming by what is termed 'intensive methods' (devilish methods in truth), where living, sentient creatures are never given normal exercise or permitted to breed offspring for their survival on earth. And yet God put his animals with such loving care, 'two of every kind' within the Ark of Noah, so that they could 'survive and multiply'.

I hope that this book will teach kinder treatment of domestic animals, in this case the *cat*. I do hope that cats will not be deprived unnaturally and cruelly of their claws, a modern development.

Here I must make a plea, to the owner of the modern domestic cat. If cats *have* to be neutered or spayed (turned into non-breeders), due to the difficulties of town life nowadays or for the convenience of their owners, then I do plead with those owners to consider allowing them to sire or kitten at least once in their lifetime so that they can survive on earth through their offspring when the time comes for them to die.

The beautiful blade of wheat gives its golden grains to the summer winds, then withers and dies, but survives a hundredfold within its grains which, when the rains of springtime come, will then grow up into new wheat plants, within each one of them the essence of the mother plant.

I plead for such survival of all our domestic animals, condemned by the surgeon's knife to lifelong sterility.

Care for cats

It is tragic for us who deeply love our cats and dogs, horses and other domestic animals that their lives are so short in length that we outlive them and have to endure the sad partings from them when old age takes them. Therefore we should make those short lives as happy, healthy and safe as possible.

'Thank God for our animals. What a blessing they are!' Those are the words of the Italian Prince of Venosa (Alberico Boncompagni Ludovisi) in a letter to me telling me of the death of a very old, beloved pointer bitch and of the agony in her eyes when she knew that she was leaving this world and her master forever, that she could no longer stay. It is unlikely that she knew, what the prince knew, that they would meet again in the kinder world beyond this one.

Remember the welcoming greetings that our animals, be it dog, cat or bird, give us on our every return home.

I particularly remember a young gypsy woman, in England's New Forest, lamenting the deaths of her parents, declaring that she had nothing any more to which to come home, not even a bird there to greet her. So I bought and gave her a bird, one bred in captivity which therefore would not suffer so much from caged life. From her I obtained the promise that the bird would be allowed to fly around within her home and we named the bird, a grey budgerigar, 'Pearlie'. The importance of animals' names is dealt with in the previous chapter of this book.

Burial of pets

My father as a college student, coming from Turkey to England, brought with him his favourite horse at a time when it was unusual for horses to travel. In very old age that horse became blind, but yet enjoyed life in a big meadow rented especially. The horse, Madralli, lived for half a century, then closed his blind eyes in eternal sleep and was buried in the meadow which had been his pleasure for so long.

I consider that burial of our pets is important. It is believed that the souls of humans and animals linger around the body for several days at least after death. It is not good to hand over the body of a beloved pet to the refuse collectors to be tossed on to some stinking refuse dump frequented by rodents. I do value pets' cemeteries and uphold that that is where the bodies of our domestic animals should be interred when death comes.

Fortunately, death for people and animals (indeed, for everything including the life of our trees and plants, which we also love) is not final. All continue to live on on earth in their substance, which is what grows up from their seed. I was once given a walnut from the Himalayas; I planted it and in several years I had a great tree in my former garden in Galilee.

Then there is 'thy likeness which is left alive'. From generation to generation the same facial features are continued, and the same sort of hair and a similar voice. There are also photographs and paintings to hold that 'likeness'.

Now I quote the beautiful lines from Shakespeare, words which give comfort when death takes away beloved ones and which apply to all living things, not only to humans.

> . . . Seed springs from seeds,
> Beauty breedeth beauty,
> And so in spite of death
> Thou dost survive in that
> Thy likeness is left alive . . .

Earlier in this chapter I have pleaded that all creatures should be allowed parenthood. 'Allowed' is a cynical word, but it does apply to the modern attitude of people to their domestic animals, in their uncaring and selfish infliction of vast numbers of cats, dogs and horses. All creatures should know the normal joy of parenthood and thus live on in their offspring.

There is also survival in names – family names handed

down from generation to generation, not just humans, but pets' names. To call a new cat by the name of its predecessor (perhaps its mother or father) brings back to mind the memory of others who have answered to that name and so keeps that memory alive.

Protection of cats

Mother cats are among the most devoted of all the domestic animals; they would lay down their lives for their kittens. Often I have heard of mother cats travelling great distances to bring back home kittens who, in some strange clairvoyant way, they knew were not in good human hands, and they have carried back the kittens in their mouths over very long distances.

Fortunately the creatures, animals and birds, have their great protectors among the saints who, though all dead long ago, are still around powerfully, in spirit.

There is the best known, St Francis of Assisi, who called the animals and birds his brothers and sisters, as he likewise called the rain, the wind, the stars, the elements.

St Hubert is a special protector of the woodland animals, the deer, the hares, the wood-doves and all the others.

El Hadr of the Arabs, the Green One, the rain-bringer, is the protector of the herds and of the eagles and the owls.

St Menas of the Greeks is also the rain-bringer and protector of the herds, of the hares, of the hawks and of sea creatures and sea birds.

My personal favourite is the demi-god Pan, whose pan-pipes I have heard in the woodlands of the world. Pan, who is half man, half goat, the beloved piper who is everywhere, freeing animals from traps and opening the doors of cages to free their inmates.

And there is further St Basil, with the fragrant, healing

basil herb named after him: Sweet Basil, *Octium basilicus*. His beautiful, pleading prayer I shall quote here and I firmly intend to include it in every new book about animals that I write henceforth. St Basil was Bishop of Caesarea in the Holy Land in AD 326. Although his prayer was given to the world when the treatment of animals was far, far less cruel than it is today, it is still a very apt piece of writing, and of everlasting Value.

O God enlarge within us the sense of fellowship with all living things, our brothers the animals – to whom Thou hast given the Earth as their home in common with us. We remember with shame that in the past we have exercised the high dominions of man with ruthless cruelty, so that the voice of the Earth, which should have gone up to Thee in song, has been a groan of suffering. May we realize that they live not for us alone, but for themselves and for Thee, and that they too love the sweetness of life.

Treatment of animals

Remember now the presentday vast slaughter of the world's wildlife, of the elephant and rhinoceros, and in the oceans the sea creatures, including the sacred dolphins, caught up in the immense dragnets of commercial fishing. Remember also the secret millions of animals of many kinds, especially cats, dogs, monkeys and sheep, used and killed by drugs and surgery in ceaseless experiments. Remember that they too loved the sweetness of life!

Even as I am writing this book, there has come along one of those ominous and pitiful situations which threatens the security of animals and which will ever be recurring so long as humans exploit their farm animals by compelling them, through hunger, to eat unnatural and often heavily-polluted foods. This is the incidence of BSE in Britain (Bovine Spongiform Encephalopathy).

All the herbivore animals have admirable skill and take great pleasure in selecting and eating leafy foods from fields, hedgerows, moorlands and other wild places. Now, however, increasing numbers of such herbivores are being compelled by their human owners to eat their own kind! They are frequently fed dried blood mixed into sawdust from slaughterhouse floors, and dried, minced-up legs and beaks of poultry, which substance is at least semi-diseased if it is taken from common battery houses that are manifold in modern poultry farming.

I have digressed, but these practices have led to this new, terrible and fatal disease affecting the brains of cattle and commonly called 'Mad Cow Disease', which has become widespread enough to result in the slaughter of vast numbers of cows and their calves. It is very distressing to think of the terror and pain these big animals have been suffering and it makes one angry because it should never have happened to these lovely and benign creatures had they only been allowed their *natural* food.

As part of the wider consequences of such unnatural practices, it has been discovered that one or more cats has died from this same cattle disease. The eating of tinned pet food is blamed, the suggestion being that some parts of diseased cattle, possibly brains, were used in pet food manufacture.

In this book there are frequent reminders to cat-owners to keep the foods of their pets natural, to prepare foods themselves, making sure that ingredient by ingredient the food is whole and not adulterated and not in any way unclean.

Now because of this threat to cats from BSE, there is fear among owners and lovers of the cat. But I can assure readers of this book that if they will take time and trouble to raise their domestic animals, cats and dogs especially, naturally, diseases will not come along to threaten and take away life.

Herbal care

Over the years I have written several books devoted to natural diet and herbal care for man and animal. If this book has pleased you, reader, I have two other herbals which should be of interest to you.

One is *The Complete Herbal Handbook for the Dog and Cat*, which gives interesting and beneficial herbal remedies for the care of dogs and cats and includes numerous testimonials of veterinary herbal cures that have been achieved by following my methods.

The other is *The Illustrated Herbal Handbook for Everyone*, which, in addition to the information about the use and remedial properties of individual herbs, has expert illustrations by Heather Wood to help in their identification. Particularly for human use.

A third herbal, *The Complete Herbal Handbook for Farm and Stable*, covers wide ground in the rearing, feeding and herbal doctoring of farm animals.

All three books have been newly revised and reissued and are published by Faber and Faber and readily available in bookshops.

Love your animals

We should love our animals deeply enough to give them daily all that they need in exercise, good meals and our friendship. The human race needs contact with the world's animals, including the cat. God put the creatures carefully and lovingly into the Ark for this purpose and instructed Noah to take into the Ark the appropriate foods for all the creatures.

As I draw near to the end of this cats' book, I am reminded by a great animal-lover especially of cats, Ruth Bouratinos of

Greece, of a quotation from that great Russian writer and prophet, Dostoevsky:

> Love the animals: God has given them the rudiments of thought and untroubled joy. Do not, therefore, trouble them, do not torture them, do not deprive them of their joy, do not go against God's intent.

Last words

Throughout history the cat has always been revered and admired. The impressive power of the domestic cat, despite its small size, caused it to be classed as a sacred animal in many parts of the world, especially in Egypt and Siam. The cat worship of the ancient Egyptians was so well known that their enemies used to take cats into war, and show them on their front lines, thus making the Egyptians hesitant to attack their foes in case they killed the cats.

In ancient times the Greeks kept weasels as pets and they were valued as very skilled mousers and having 'pretty' ways. The reason that weasels were kept as pets was because export of cats from Egypt was strictly banned as cats in Egypt were sacred.

Modern man has no right to misuse for human 'convenience' this sacred animal, the domestic cat. All who own a cat or cats agree that the essence of this animal is in its eyes – those night-seeing orbs, which glint and flash wonderfully in night's darkness, like the tiger! It is interesting that those illuminating studs used on roads to guide motorists by night are called 'cats' eyes'.

Cats' eyes look into those of mankind and warn: 'O man, do not trample on my rights. Remove my claws perhaps.' We agree. Cats' green eyes flash, and man is cautioned and maybe shamed. This is how I see those eyes:

CATS' EYES

Cats' eyes! Green! Green!
A-dazzle, a-glint, alight,
In the night. Oh! tiger-bright!

Cats' eyes! Green! Green!
Stealers of the emerald's gleam,
And the halcyon's sheen.

Cats' eyes! Green! Green!
Eyes that tantalize,
Bewitch and mesmerize!

Cats' eyes! Green! Green!
Foes of evil rat and mouse,
Lured by eyes from hidden house!

Cats' eyes! Green! Green!
Sharers of the owl's keen sight.
Both keep watch through every night.

Cats' eyes! Green! Green!
Ye bold captains of moonlight
Flash your emeralds in the night.
Oh! Cats' eyes! Green! Green!

Juliette de Baïracli Levy

7

The Herbs in this Book

Common wild plants, Garden Plants and Herbs, Herbs to be purchased from sellers, Prepared herbal products, Some herbal suppliers

Common wild plants

BILBERRY, WHORTLEBERRY (*Vaccinium myrtillus*. Vacciniaceae) Found on boggy heaths and on mountainsides. Its edible berries are well known.

BLACKBERRY, BRAMBLE (*Rubus fructicosus*. Rosaceae) A common thorny hedgerow and wasteland herb, known for its juicy and edible fruits.

BORAGE (*Borago officinalis*. Boraginaceae) Field and woodland, distinguished by its rough leaves and intensely blue flowers.

BROOM (*Cytisus scoparius*. Leguminosae) Found on dry heaths and sandy soils. Possesses yellow, pea-form flowers.

CHAMOMILE (*Anthemis nobilis*. Compositae) Waste places and damp places. Fragrant, small, daisy-like flowers; very scented, feathery leaves.

CHICKWEED (*Stellaria media*, Caryophyllaceae) A tiny pasture herb with white, starry flowers.

CLOVER (Red) (*Trifolium pratense*. Leguminosae) A plant of pastures, with trefoil leaves and globes of red flowers.

COMFREY (*Symphytum officinale*. Boraginaceae) Inhabits ditchsides, though will also grow in dry places. Now often cultivated as a fodder crop especially in Russia. Large, rough leaves; pinkish or creamy bell-like flowers.

DANDELION (*Taraxacum officinale*. Compositae) Common weed found on waste ground, on banks, and in gardens. Composite bright yellow flowers.

DOCK (*Rumex sanguineus*. Polygonaceae) A common broad-leaf weed, with spikes of loose, rusty-coloured, reed-like flowers.

ELDER, ELDERBERRY (*Sambucus nigra*. Caprifoliaceae) A small tree or shrub, with rich-scented, flat heads of creamy flowers, producing edible black berries.

ELDER, DWARF or GROUND (*Sambucus ebulus*. Caprifoliaceae) Grows in waste places, is also a persistent garden weed. Resembles a small elder, but its leaves have a stronger colour and its flowers are scentless.

GOOSE-GRASS, CLEAVERS (*Galium aparine*. Rubiaceae) A trailing weed with round fruits and square stems, both of clinging nature.

GREATER CELANDINE (*Chelidonium majus*. Papaveraceae) Found by old walls and on rubble, also outskirts of woods. Grey leaves and small, frail, yellow flowers which shed their petals very easily.

HOLLY (*Ilex aquifolium*. Aquifoliaceae) A well-known red-berried bush or tree with prickly leaves.

HOREHOUND (*Marrubium vulgare*. Labiatae) Common in woodland and in hedgerows. Greyish, slightly woolly leaves; spikes of colourless flowers.

IVY (*Hedera helix*. Araliaceae) A well-known evergreen climbing plant with colourless, sweet-scented blossoms. Found on trees, banks, old walls, etc.

MALE FERN (*Aspidium filix-mas*. Filices) Likes woods and shady banks. Distinguished by its tall fern foliage which has numerous scales on the under surface of leaves, and bears brown spores.

MARSH-MALLOW (*Althea officinalis*. Malvaceae) Of waysides, pink flowers, very round, dark foliage.

MEADOWSWEET (*Filipendula ulmaria*. Rosaceae) Grows in wet meadows. Has rose-form leaves, plumes of creamy, sweet-scented flowers.

NETTLE, STINGING NETTLE (*Urtica dioicia*. Urticaceae) A tall perennial, known by its leaves which sting sharply.

OAK (*Quercus robur*. Loganiaceae) A tree of woodlands. Has notable oval fruits in green cups, called acorns.

PLANTAIN (*Plantago major*. Plantaginaceae) Of pastureland and waste places. Distinguished by its flat-growing, oval-shaped and ribbed leaves, and unusual flowering spike, resembling a small bulrush, of greenish-brown hue.

RASPBERRY (*Rubus idaeus*. Rosaceae) A bramble-like woodland shrub, known for its juicy red berries.

THYME (*Thymus serpyllum*. Labiatae) Of moorland and sunny banks. Tiny leaves, the tufts of white-pink flowers of very sweet and aromatic scent.

TOAD-FLAX (*Linaria vulgaris*. Scrophulariaceae) Of pastures and waste places, distinguished by its yellow and cream 'snap-dragon' shaped flowers.

VIOLET (Sweet) (*Viola odorata*. Violaceae) Of shady banks and woodlands. Well known by its fragrant purple flowers. The garden species is also used.

WATERCRESS (*Nasturtium officinale*. Cruciferae) Well-known wild salad plant, growing in running streams, especially spring-water streams. If shop-bought, take care that it does not come from still, copper-sulphate water.

WILD ROSE, SWEET BRIAR (*Rosa* species. Rosaceae) A well-known shrub of hedgerow and woodland. Distinguished by its sweet-scented pink flowers and hard, red, shiny, edible fruits – 'hips'.

WOOD SAGE (*Teucrium scorodonia*. Labiatae) Of shady places and woodlands. Rough, dark leaves, spiky, greenish-yellow, hooded flowers.

YARROW (*Achillea millefolium*. Compositae) A weed of lawns and pastures. Feathery leaves, flat heads of composite, tiny rose or cream-coloured flowers.

Garden plants and herbs

ASPARAGUS (*Asparagus officinalis*. Liliaceae) Known for its edible shoots. Also found wild.

BALM (*Melissa officinalis*. Labiatae) Hairy leaves, whorls of creamy, hooded flowers: much sought by bees.

CRESS, GARDEN CRESS (*Lepidium sativum*. Cruciferae) The common salad herb with 'hot' leaves.

GARLIC (*Allium* species. Liliaceae) Easily grown in gardens or bought from greengrocers. The wild variety grows in damp woodland and pastures.

HOLLYHOCK (*Althea rosea*. Malvaceae) Well known for its tallness and large flowers of various colours with squarish petals.

HYSSOP (*Hyssopus officinalis*. Labiate) An attractive, very aromatic border plant. Much celebrated in the Bible.

LAVENDER (*Lavandula vera*. Labiatae) Well known, very fragrant when dry or fresh, has small greyish leaves and spikes of blue flowers.

LILY OF THE VALLEY (*Convallaria majalis*. Liliaceae) Well-known for its sweet-scented, white flowers; much planted in gardens.

MARIGOLD (*Calendula officinalis*. Compositae) The well-known hardy annual of bright, orange-hued, daisy form or double daisy flowers.

MARJORAM (*Origanum vulgare* or *onites*. Labiatae) Very aromatic, of mountain origin, and resembles a tall, wild thyme.

MINT (*Mentha viridis*. Labiatae)   The common garden salad plant with mint scent.

MUSTARD (Black) (*Brassica nigra*. Cruciferae)   A common garden weed, with bright yellow flowers and strong-tasting cress-like leaves.

PARSLEY (*Petroselinum crispum*. Umbelliferae)   Common garden salad herb, with flat or tightly curled leaves of intense green.

PEONY (*Paeonia officinalis*. Ranunculaceae)   It has distinct solitary red or pink, large, many petalled flowers, and large, fringed, leaves.

POPPY (OPIUM) and WILD, RED (*Papaver somniferum* and *Papaver rhoeas*. Papaveraceae)   The former is a tall plant with grey-blue foliage and big, white-cream flowers; the latter, small, hairy stemmed, with small, brilliant red flowers.

RASPBERRY (see Common wild plants, p. 130)

ROSEMARY (*Rosmarinus officinalis*. Labiatae)   A very aromatic plant of grey-green foliage and small, hooded light blue flowers.

RUE (*Ruta graveolens*. Rutaceae)   Distinguished by its much-divided flat, greyish leaves, and small yellow flowers of bitter scent.

SAGE (*Salvia officinalis*. Labiatae)   Popular garden culinary herb, also grows in abundance wild, on hills and plains. Grey, strongly scented foliage; spikes of blue flowers.

Herbs to be purchased from sellers

ELM (SLIPPERY) or RED ELM (*Ulmus rubra*. Ulmaceae)   The pink-hued, very aromatic bark is famous for its medicinal properties.

EUCALYPTUS (*Eucalyptus globulus*. Myrtaceae)   The extracted oil most used in veterinary medicine, has to be purchased. Leaves and bark can be gathered from the tree.

FENUGREEK (SEED) (*Trigonella foenum-graecum*. Leguminosae) The seed, except in Egypt and Tunisia, has to be purchased.

LIQUORICE (*Glycyrrhiza glabra*. Leguminosae) The root can be bought from herbalists or the black solid juice, usually called Spanish liquorice and sold in sticks.

QUASSIA CHIPS A very bitter wood from a shrub. Purchased finely flaked, and used as an insecticide, especially for lice. Can be ordered from herbal suppliers.

SENNA (*Cassia acutifolia*. Leguminosae) The foliage and flat seed-pods are sold by most herbalists and drug stores. The flat seeds are the part used mostly as a powerful laxative.

SKULLCAP (*Scutellaria galericulata*. Labiatae) The plant grows wild in Europe and North America, but is not widely distributed. In some parts it is rare. The dried herb is procurable from most herbalists.

WITCH HAZEL (*Hamamelis virginiana*. Hamamelidaceae) The bark is sold by herbalists, also its extract in alcohol. Most drug stores sell this famed astringent and antiseptic extract.

PREPARED HERBAL PRODUCTS

Prepared herbal products are becoming increasingly hard to obtain and to use with confidence. The main problem is that destructive modernity has moved into herbs and is likely to remain because herbs have become 'big business'.

Formerly, all supplies of herbs were natural products. They were in the hands of true herbalists only, devoted gatherers who carefully air-dried herbs in their own skilled ways.

Few herbs are gathered presentday from the wild places of the world as they once were. Modern developments are cutting down the number of places for wild flowers to grow and in some countries, such as the United Kingdom, there are government restrictions on uprooting and picking of wild plants. In addition herbs are being grown by the acre for commercial gain and are then dried by electricity. Quick heat-drying turns the herbs an unnatural bright colour and makes them very brittle, but the greatest harm done is that the vital medicinal part of herbs, the essential oils, are lost, having evaporated, leaving the herbs almost worthless so far as their medicinal properties are concerned.

Frequently I have purchased herbs by post and found them useless to me. A recent purchase of French lavender – and France is famed for this herb – was entirely without any lavender fragrance at all. It was therefore thrown out for compost in my garden!

So one needs to be very careful concerning commercial products nowadays: are they being made from worthless herbs, ruined by commercial growing and drying? Some of my former suppliers have broken faith with me in the past and with followers of my work who needed the products I had advised. Some have even dared to add chemicals to my recommended treatments; this was done in the USA for my vital treatment for heartworms.

If you do see persons advertising that they are selling *my* formulae, I advise you, if possible, to take a look at their premises before becoming a client and see what they themselves are like and what sort of herbs they are using and selling, of natural or unnatural quality. When visiting reputable firms in the past I have surprised them in the midst of having their premises sprayed with insecticides, the herbs in storage there not being protected from contact with the spray.

If herbal products cannot be obtained by post with confidence, then learn to make home remedies. One does not want one's animals to be deprived of herbal help because people are exploiting herbs for mere commercial gain.

Basic advice for home-made remedies is not to use the very potent herbs, which do need careful prescribing. Instead, substitute with milder ones. Rue and wormwood are both very potent: so omit rue, which can be replaced by vervain or marjoram, and ditto wormwood, which can be replaced by the milder southernwood (of the same family). Rue and wormwood can be used safely externally. Amounts then do not matter and both are great herbs.

Here are some simple basic aids for Natural Rearing which can be home-made; no precise formula is necessary.

For external use to deter skin parasites and to treat wounds and skin ailments: wormwood or southernwood, rue, rosemary, eucalyptus and pink bark, sage, rosemary, all in dried powder form.

For internal use for infectious ailments and worms: equal parts of southernwood, sage garlic, a few spice cloves, made into pills with flour and thick honey as a base.

To wean young animals of all kinds and to nourish sick ones: grind flaked barley in a handmill to make into barley flour and to every cupful of this flour add a tablespoon of powdered slippery elm bark and several teaspoons of powdered flaked rye plus one teaspoon of powdered almond kernels. Make into a paste with honey, then add several spoonfuls of hot water (not so hot as to kill the life in the honey). Finally, add to the paste half a pint of warm milk, fresh milk, if possible, and unpasteurized, but *not* so-called long-life milk or tinned or dried milk. The flaking of the barley renders it digestible and no cooking is needed, merely the soaking in milk during the making of the complete mixture. Give as much of this mixture as the young animal needs to take in order to satisfy its appetite.

Natural minerals supplement

As a daily tonic: seaweed in powder form, the green leaves finely cut. To every tablespoon of powdered seaweed add one teaspoon of finely-minced leaves of parsley, chickweed, fennel or dill, clover, dandelion, nasturtium, cress, mint. Mix well and sprinkle a tablespoon into the food once daily. For the seaweed use deep-sea kelp to guard against the seashore pollution of seaweeds. Use as much variety as possible in the leaves.

SOME HERBAL SUPPLIERS

My advice is that it is best to deal with the really big herbal firms, many years established and with a good reputation to maintain, and to make sure that the herbs they sell you have not been spoilt (deprived of their essential oils by machine-drying). Or find local herbalists who dry their herbs carefully at home.

Better still, grow your own herbs so that you can gather them fresh from your garden or window box and air-dry them yourself, as described in Chapter 4.

Recommended suppliers

Larkhall Natural Health plc, of Forest Road, Charlbury, Oxford OX3 3HH, England, supply some of my herbal formulae and my books. (They are not licensed for the USA.)

The Fiddes Paynes sell dried herbs and my herbal books at The Spice Warehouse, Pepper Alley, Banbury, Oxfordshire, England.

Culpeper shops, now in many towns, usually stock good quality herbs in dry form, also in prepared mixtures.

Postscript

I sincerely regret that it is no longer possible to answer readers' veterinary problems sent to me in the post. Because I travel so much, months often go by without mail reaching me and very many letters are lost as a result of my being out of reach of mail.

To make sure that the treatments for ailments I have given in this book can all be followed with ease, I have looked at them closely to make sure that no help will be needed from myself.

Of course there are many ailments not dealt with in this book, as I wrote earlier. To have included them all would have made it a quite different book, no more a useful handbook.

If I were to answer all the letters I receive, I should be writing letters all day and all night. Impossible! Nor can I, in fairness, answer a few chosen people and not answer all. Unjust. Again impossible!

From early childhood I have had a deep love for animals, and now that I have reached the usual age of retirement from work, I know that I can best serve animals by practical study of their needs in the field, during my continuing travels, and not monotonously, and *unwillingly*, confined to a room with a typewriter.

Therefore, please do not write to me. I thank you for reading this book and I know that it will help your cats as it has mine.

Juliette de Baïracli Levy

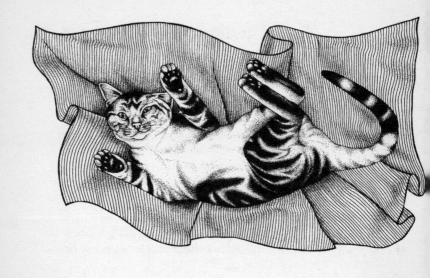

Index